Why Millions Died

Before the War on Infectious Diseases

George H. Scherr

UNIVERSITY PRESS OF AMERICA,® INC.
Lanham • Boulder • New York • Toronto • Plymouth, UK

Copyright © 2012 by
University Press of America,® Inc.
4501 Forbes Boulevard
Suite 200
Lanham, Maryland 20706
UPA Acquisitions Department (301) 459-3366

Estover Road
Plymouth PL6 7PY
United Kingdom

Library of Congress Control Number: 2011927068
ISBN: 978-0-7618-5555-2 (paperback : alk. paper)
eISBN: 978-0-7618-5556-9

In memory of Rita,
the mother of my children

Knowledge after the
event is always easy, and
problems once solved present
no difficulties, indeed, may be
represented as never having
had any. . . .

—Justice Joseph McKenna

Contents

Illustrations

FIGURES

TABLES

Preface

In 1951, I was appointed Assistant Professor of Microbiology at the Creighton University School of Medicine in Omaha, Nebraska. In 1953, I was awarded a research grant from the United States Navy to study the pathogenesis of various infectious diseases. I presented a paper at the 6th International Congress of Microbiology in Rome in September 1953, flying there aboard a military plane courtesy of the United States Navy.

Specially reprinted documents of distinguished Italian microbiologists were passed out to members of the Congress. In addition, all attendees at the meeting received a special postage stamp issued by the Italian government in honor of the Congress.

En route back to the United States in a military transport plane, I went through my briefcase and reviewed the various data I had accumulated at the meeting. I discovered the stamp prepared by the Italian government which showed a picture of a person identified as Agostino Bassi. Since I had never heard of him, I asked some of my associates on the plane who had attended the meeting if they had ever heard of him. They said they had never heard of him either. It piqued my curiosity that a presumably distinguished microbiologist named Agostino Bassi was literally unknown to many of the microbiologists who had attended the meeting. When the opportunity presented itself, I went to the Library of Congress to look up Agostino Bassi. I discovered that he had worked in Pavia in the early part of the 19th century, graduated from the University of Pavia in Italy as a lawyer, but then altered his interest to diseases, especially the disease that was devastating the silkworm industry in Italy and in France.

Over the years, I traveled to the University of Pavia and was received by the library staff and permitted to copy some of the old documents that were in their files describing the research of Agostino Bassi. I discovered that the research work of Bassi and the conclusions he had drawn clearly justified the consideration that he had been the first to characterize the role of infectious microorganisms as the etiological agents of disease. In studying the work of other microbiologists that had worked during the studies of Bassi, I further learned of the nefarious role that Louis Pasteur played in repeating the work of Bassi and claiming for himself the privilege of being the first to elaborate the germ theory of disease, thirty years after Bassi had published all of his work. I also discovered other evidence of Pasteur's fraudulent activities which were revealed only after all of his research notebooks were laid open to the public contrary to his wishes as set forth in his will.

The adversaries who rejected the idea that microorganisms could cause these deadly infections and the delay in implementing those measures that would prevent or treat many of the epidemics that raged, resulted in infections that devastated millions of people until the idea of microbial infections causing diseases became universally accepted.

George H. Scherr, Ph.D.

Acknowledgments

It is not possible to achieve any semblance of success without the encourage-ment of many people from all walks of life who labor alongside you and pave the way for your aspirations to take shape and materialize.

My teachers from the very first grade to my advanced degrees were excep-tional in expending their time and efforts to provide a favorable climate so that students could enjoy and prosper from their education. I was fortunate to grow up in New York City during the mayoral tenure of Fiorello H. La Guardia. He ordered that entertainment be provided without cost to the people of New York City. He even provided performers from the Metropolitan Opera House to go to schools and entertain 4th and 5th grade students.

Skill and patience in organizing and maintaining the vast amount of ref-erences that had to be reviewed in order to compile the data in the course of history presented here is deserving of the efforts of only one person—Ms. Jean Jacobs.

Multiple reviews of the entire manuscript and placing it in a grammatical state deserving of the English language were achieved by the scholarship and perseverance of Mr. Dale Jacobs.

The library work of Dr. Claude Regnier in Paris, France, in identifying the Chamberland patents is very much appreciated.

I should also like to acknowledge with appreciation the permission to re-produce the drawings of the experiments of Spallanzani prepared by the Kent School District in Kent, Washington.

I acknowledge with appreciation the consideration of the Welcome Foun-dation for its courtesy in permitting us to reproduce the painting of "The Cow-Pock" in the chapter relative to Edward Jenner.

I must single out particularly Professor Robert Weaver at the University of Kentucky whose good humor, patient disposition, and friendly nature made possible my graduate degrees.

My dear friend and colleague, the late Professor Max Rafelson at the University of Illinois School of Medicine, provided a model of what a brilliant scholar, humane individual, and nobility of purpose he exemplified; where all of these attributes are rarely found in one individual.

I want to extend my sincere appreciation to the library staff at the University of Pavia School of Medicine for their courtesies in providing me with access to historical documents and books showing the history of the distinguished scientists who were on the staff of the medical school. Also, my gratitude is expressed for permitting me to procure pertinent copies of those documents.

I am deeply indebted to my wife, Marge, for her patience, perseverance, and support for my literary efforts.

The review of the entire manuscript and the multiple suggestions provided by my daughter Lisa, which served to improve the clarity of this document, are very much appreciated.

Finally, above all, I am indebted to my late wife, Rita, whose confidence shown by her thoughts and actions in supporting my efforts never wavered; her devotion to scholarship acted as a model impetus for our three children, all of whom would make any parent proud.

Introduction

The scientist is predominantly preoccupied with the concept of "discovery." However, mere discovery of a novel idea, mathematical theorem, or biological concept, in and of itself, may lack the scientist's understanding of the significance of what has been discovered. There have also been cases of investigators who learn of discoveries previously achieved by other individuals who may not have the prestige nor the capability, for one reason or another, to capitalize on their discovery, and their work is adopted by the more aggressive investigators and claimed as their own. An excellent example is the discovery of the double helix of DNA.

Thus James Watson and Francis Crick may well argue that the radio-diffraction photograph achieved by Rosalind Franklin at Cambridge demonstrated the double helix of DNA, but that Franklin was not cognizant of the significance of what lay on her table until it was removed without her permission and placed into the hands of Watson and Crick, who recognized its importance. Whether such a conclusion is an honest one or self-serving has been debated in a detailed analysis by Brenda Maddox documenting the course of events of the discovery of the double helix in her book *Rosalind Franklin—The Dark Lady of DNA*. It was clear that Rosalind Franklin was a brilliant investigator in her own right, and was working in a man's world under conditions, due to her bout with cancer, that did not afford her the opportunity to capitalize on her discovery. It also remains clear that the radio-image prepared by Franklin was improperly removed from her office and turned over to Watson and Crick, who then went on to claim the discovery of the double helix. What turned out to be even more egregious for these claims is that the authors attempted to denigrate the capabilities and the social standing of Franklin by writing about her efforts in a derogatory vein. It took the revelations of Brenda Maddox in researching the entire course of events to correct what was a misguided credit that omitted the research of Rosalind Franklin as the first demonstration of the double helix.

Discovery of a novel concept may also languish for many years before its practical application can be achieved by investigators who more readily recognize the significance of the discovery. One such example is the discovery by Alexander Fleming in 1929 of the inhibition of a *Staphylococcus* culture growing on a Petri dish, where a mold accidentally got into the plate due to the lack of total exclusion of contaminants. Fleming noticed that the mold growing on the plate reduced the growth of the *Staphylococci* around the mold, thus indicating that something in the mold, presumably an antibiotic, may be inhibiting the growth of the *Staphylococcus* organism. Various investigations and studies were necessary before the antibiotic could be produced commercially and applied where applicable to certain microorganisms that would be susceptible to penicillin. These included studies to investigate the means of producing penicillin in quantity, studies on its potential toxicity for the human when injected in various amounts, and studies to determine which infectious diseases penicillin might be effective against. It took approximately eleven years after the discovery by Fleming before practical applications and experimental studies with the culture of *Penicillium notatum* showed that it produced an antibiotic, penicillin, which could safely be used to treat infectious diseases.

In the mid-1800's, Gregor Mendel, a botanist and monk living and working in a monastery in Austria, discovered that the colors of peas would differentiate themselves in ratios that would follow certain genetic laws. Mendel's discovery languished for approximately fifty years until in 1900, Hugo deVries in the Netherlands, Erich Tschermak von Seysenegg in Austria, and Carl Correns in Germany rediscovered Mendelian genetics. It is not clear whether any of the three investigators knew of Mendel's work or, in fact, whether any one of the three was cognizant of the work being done by the other two. The idea, therefore, that discovery may be achieved by two or three independent workers may depend on the course of events and the development in their respective fields where sufficient knowledge has been gleaned to make it feasible to pursue studies that would lead to the same conclusion and end results.

Under some circumstances, two or more independent scientists may give radically different explanations for the end results of similar research. Thus Professor Augustine Branigan in her excellent treatise on *The Social Basis of Scientific Discoveries* points out that three scientists simultaneously, but independently, discovered "fire air" (oxygen)—Joseph Priestley of England, Antoine Lavoisier of France, and Carl Wilhelm Scheele of Sweden. Both Priestley and Lavoisier in the late 1700's isolated a gas and confirmed the presence of this gas in air, which we now characterize as oxygen; but they ascribed different explanations for what they had discovered. Priestley considered the oxygen as "dephlogisticated air," and Lavoisier understood it as a principle of combustion that was produced only when the oxygen united with heat.

Although other researchers such as Hales, Black, Vayen, and Scheele produced pure oxygen, they generally all had different understandings of what oxygen was and its significance.

Another attribute that clouds the authenticity of discovery concerns the utilization of hindsight. As the distinguished jurist Joseph McKenna once said: "Knowledge after the event is always easy, and problems once solved present no difficulties, indeed, may be represented as never having had any. . . ."

Thus, almost every patent office in the world usually challenges the validity of a patent application by pointing out that the novel combination of a structure A and a structure B as claimed by an inventor as producing a novel device hitherto not previously discovered is merely a development of the fact that A has been well-demonstrated by one investigator to be novel and B was shown by another investigator to be novel, and that anyone working in the field would have the common sense to combine A and B and claim a unique product. With that logic being extended to all inventions, one might well close down most of the patent offices in the world. Even Thomas Edison's patent demonstrating the performance of an incandescent lamp might well have been rejected today on the basis of the fact that sending electricity through a wire would permit it to glow red and increasing the electric current going through the wire would make the wire glow even brighter. Concomitantly, it had been known for over a hundred years that burning requires the presence of oxygen. Therefore, with these two well-known observations, merely putting a wire in a glass bulb and evacuating the air, which excludes the oxygen, and then sending current through that wire to make it glow is not a novel idea, since any investigator would have thought of it.

In the main square of Grenoble, France, a monument to Monsieur Luminaire credits him with being the first person to invent the incandescent light bulb. Yet outside of the French community and in the minds of many scientists, it is Edison who has been credited with being the first to invent the electric light bulb. This is probably due to the fact that he immediately saw the application for the incandescent lamp in lighting up entire communities and began to apply his invention to that end as quickly as possible.

Erroneous conclusions by scientific investigators have not been uncommon. Some of the conclusions have been deliberately contrived; others may have been inadvertently arrived at due to preconceived notions of the investigator and are inconsistent with the facts if otherwise examined by a more objective investigator.

A misunderstanding of the scientific approach and its inherent variations of application has made it difficult to characterize science as an attribute of study that would be followed by all those investigating natural problems. An excellent analysis of the scientific approach has been presented by Carlo Lastrucci in his study *The Scientific Approach*.

Thus, data published by Samuel George Morton in 1830 concluded that the cranial capacity of different groups of people was largest among Caucasians, followed by American Indians, and then by African people. The conclusion was drawn that the largest mean cranial capacity also meant a higher IQ. A review of the data showed that there was no mean difference between any of these groups and that Morton's conclusions were arrived at, not by a deliberate manipulation of data, but due to unconscious inconsistencies and miscalculations that drove him to the conclusions he made.

A more flagrant perversion of the facts was achieved by Dr. Summerlin, who was engaged in studies to achieve the transplantation of tissue from one species to another. Following a substantial research grant, a search committee from the National Institutes of Health arrived at the premises to discuss his grant renewal. While coming down in the elevator with a caged white rat, Dr. Summerlin removed a felt-tipped pen from his coat. He then planted a black patch on this white rat, for which he ultimately claimed a successful transplantation from a species of black rat to a white one.

The attending group was most impressed, following which he asked one of the dieners to take the rat back to the animal room. The animal room was being washed and cleaned at that time, and the diener discovered that the black mark was beginning to run. The revelation, which ultimately made its way to the director of the Sloan-Kettering Institute, raised a question as to why this had been done. The answer was that he felt that he was very close to achieving the result and needed a little more time and research grant money to solve the problem. See *False Prophets* by Alexander Kohn (1986).

Chapter One

Historical

The various practices of how to deal with serious diseases and injuries over the centuries have been well documented by many historians. Many of the ancient recommendations were primarily based on ideas that were supernatural in origin. The observations that large beetles could emanate from animal dung led the Egyptians to believe in the spontaneous origin of life, a concept that was fairly ubiquitous up until the middle of the 19th century.

The organized practice of medicine may have originated with Imhotep, who lived about 2650 B.C. Imhotep became regarded as the Egyptian God of Medicine. The Greeks identified him with the Greek God Aesculapius, their God of Healing. The Egyptian practice of medicine was markedly enlarged by the Hebrews. They developed a wide literature, not only dealing with diseased states, but also providing information on social and personal hygiene that was to significantly improve the prevention of infectious diseases. However, the understanding of the origin of infectious diseases still required a long time before it could be promulgated and accepted. In the first two centuries B.C., there was no uniform education for "doctors" to heal the sick and the injured. It was not uncommon to lay sick or injured people in the streets so that anyone passing by who might have knowledge of how to cope with the disease or injury could offer some advice. This was fairly prevalent during the Babylonian Era.

Long before Van Leeuwenhoek recorded his first observations of microscopic life, there had been philosophical mutterings about the possible existence of living things that are invisible to the naked eye, as seen in Figure 1.1. In part, some of these speculations arose from the logical conclusions drawn by a number of Greek philosophers. They postulated that it is possible to take a piece of bread or meat and keep cutting it into smaller and smaller pieces, and still have bread or meat. Therefore, it should be possible for pieces to be

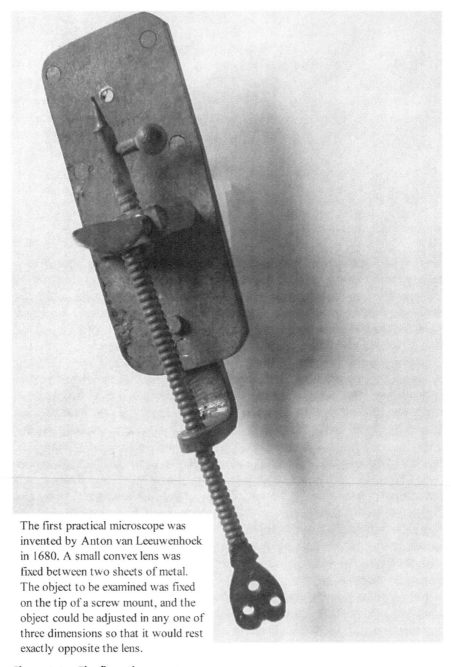

The first practical microscope was
invented by Anton van Leeuwenhoek
in 1680. A small convex lens was
fixed between two sheets of metal.
The object to be examined was fixed
on the tip of a screw mount, and the
object could be adjusted in any one of
three dimensions so that it would rest
exactly opposite the lens.

Figure 1.1.   The first microscope.

cut so small that they are invisible to the naked eye and still constitute all of the attributes of bread or meat.

Even Aristotle postulated that there might be certain diseases which cause contagion that are invisible, but obviously there was no way that such a determination could be proven during his time. Hippocrates described white patches that occurred in patients, which we now know to have been the cause of candidiasis (moniliasis). The Romans recognized the ringworm lesions in patients. However, they attributed them to insect bites and did not have the resources to identify them as being caused by superficial mycotic organisms (dermatophytes). They called these infections *tinea*, meaning small insect larvae. The term is still utilized as a description of the superficial dermatophyte infections.

The Greeks recognized these superficial dermatophyte infections, but characterized them as *Herpes* (from the Greek word *to creep*) because of the tendency of the rash to occur in circular forms; again a term which has survived centuries of development in clinical microbiology, but is now used specifically to refer to viral organisms of a specific etiological type.

As early as the latter part of the 16th century, the Swiss physician Paracelsus insisted that there must be invisible organisms that cause disease, again without the ability to provide proof or documentation.

The Chinese for many centuries had accumulated a considerable repertoire of treatments utilizing various herbs and extracts of plants, and this grew to an enormous 52-volume pharmacopoeia in the 16th century. In fact, the utilization of an oil being used for leprosy was developed by the Chinese in the 14th century. Chaulmoogra oil continued to be used up to the 19th century for the treatment of leprosy in all of the western countries. Extracts from various plants, such as castor oil, Cannabis from Indian hemp, and an extract from an herb from which ephedrine was extracted, had been used by the Chinese for approximately 4,000 years. In fact, ephedrine is still being used for the treatment of asthma and related conditions. What was essentially forbidden was the utilization of dead bodies; hence any knowledge of anatomy was due to the accidental discovery of people that might have been attacked by wild dogs and killed. This provided some information of the anatomy up to about the last part of the 14th century.

Despite the fact that there were no microscopes or an understanding of the germ theory of disease for hundreds of years, the Chinese had practiced the inoculation of a small amount of matter isolated from a smallpox lesion. The inoculation resulted in a mild state of the disease, and insured a state of immunity against future exposure to smallpox. It was practiced for centuries until, in 1796, the British physician Edward Jenner observed that milkmaids often contracted cowpox—minor lesions that resembled smallpox but were much less deadly. Concomitantly, he discovered that these women were immune to smallpox, which was prevalent in England and other countries on the continent. As a result of these observations, Jenner used cowpox to inoculate people, which served as an immunological preventative for smallpox disease exposure.

The early Hindus believed that the body contained a series of elementary (chemical) substances and that these in the right proportion constituted the healthy blood, flesh, fat, bone, marrow, bile, and semen. The Hindus also believed that semen could be produced from all parts of the body and not from any individual part or organ.

With the advent of the 14th and 15th centuries, Italy became a significant impetus for the motivation of research and development in the field of medicine. The almost uniform prohibition against dissection of the human body throughout Europe and Asia was slowly being lifted. One of the first major efforts to understand the human anatomy was undertaken by Mondino dei Liucci (or Raimondino de Liuzzi), who was born in Bologna about 1270 and received a medical degree at the University of Bologna in 1290. His first dissection in 1350 was performed at the University of Bologna. Mondino's continued studies of the human anatomy ultimately resulted in the publishing of the first manual of anatomy, *Anothomia*, in 1316.[1] This monumental and extraordinary publication contained no illustrations! However, it became the guideline and universally accepted treatise on the anatomy of the human body. In fact, Mondino's treatise, written by his own hand in Latin, utilized many of the Arabic terms that had originated with Galen for the abdominal walls—the peritoneum—as well as other parts of the body.

In 1543, Andreas Vesalius, a professor of anatomy at the University of Padua, published a seminal volume "on the structure of the human body" based on dissections that he had performed. His investigations had improved the understanding of the role of veins and arteries in the human body. These studies at Padua were then followed up by Gabriel Fallopius and again by Hieronymous Fabricius of Aquapendente, whose important work on the valves of the veins was published in 1603. The works of these three anatomists provided the basis for William Harvey's revolutionary theory on the circulation of the blood, the observations of which have remained essentially valid to this day.

A treatise by the Venetian scholar Girolamo Fracastoro in the early part of the 16th century postulated that syphilis and tuberculosis were caused by invisible living organisms which were able to multiply and cause disease. As a corollary of these deliberations, prostitutes were supervised to avoid transmission of syphilis, but the understanding of hygiene as is currently practiced was nonexistent.

The investigations by the German scholar Athanasius Kircher in the mid-1600's, although recognizing that there may be a contagious element for the disease called *pest* at that time, never clarified the organism or the concept of contagion. Utilizing a microscope available at the time, Kircher examined the pus of *buboes* (swollen lymph glands) from victims that had contracted the plague. He, with some reluctance, attributed to these bodies the possible agents that caused the disease and called the bodies *minima animalcula*.

Christian Lange working in 1761 reported an epidemic of skin diseases, but again lacked the tools to characterize the disease as being caused by microorganisms. He suggested that there might be such minute organisms that could be responsible for this epidemic disease of the skin. Lange also characterized measles and smallpox and a number of other diseases of infants and children as being caused by live organisms, but he was unable to identify them or to characterize these diseases as being contagious.

A number of investigators shared the opinions and observations of Lange, again without being able to characterize the organisms or elaborate the concept of microorganisms causing contagious diseases, such as Purcell, Siegler, and Pollini in 1685.

It was the development of the microscope by Anton van Leeuwenhoek in the mid-1600's that opened the door to observing this invisible hoard of organisms and made it possible for investigators to experiment and identify the various organisms that might be responsible for a disease. Van Leeuwenhoek's microscope had a magnification that could bring into view small insects and microorganisms, especially molds and yeasts.

Although Van Leeuwenhoek was able to observe and record many microorganisms invisible to the naked eye, he never did elucidate the opinion that they could be responsible for diseases of man and animals. In 1680, Van Leeuwenhoek described and drew the microorganisms present in the tartar of his teeth as well as brewers' yeasts. He was thus the first person to have described microbes.

With the availability of microscopy and the gradual improvement of the magnification of microscopes, the German physician Johann Elsholtz in 1679 attributed to small organisms the possible causative agents of numerous infectious diseases.

In 1687, Giovan Cosimo Bonomo and Giacinto Cestoni discovered and characterized the acarus worm as being responsible for scabies, or "the itch" as it was known at that time. These observations strengthened the opinions of other workers as to the parasitic origin of many diseases. This doctrine was liberally promoted in France by Andre in 1700 and also by Harsuckle in 1730. At about the same time, a group of Italian investigators, such as Francesco

Redi, Lansizzi, and Valacineric, liberally supported the concept that microscopic organisms could cause infectious diseases.

In the 1700's, the Swedish naturalist, Carolus Linnaeus, had recorded in his massive tome *Systema Naturae* all of the known organisms, including small ones of the genus *chaos.* In 1757, however, he admitted that there were exceedingly small organisms, and some perhaps not yet discovered or well known, which could be the cause of contagious diseases, including venereal diseases.

Because yeasts and molds and microscopic parasites could readily be observed with the magnification of the primitive microscope developed by Van Leeuwenhoek, many workers and scholars in the field, including Van Leeuwenhoek, concluded that the microscopic organisms which cause fermentation and putrefaction are essentially one and the same.[2] Numerous detractors opposed the concept that microscopic organisms were the etiological agents of disease.

Yet there was a gradual increase in interest and observations—and gradually in organized experimental research, primarily encouraged by Lazzaro Spallanzani at the University of Pavia—which encouraged a resurgence of interest in the concept that germs caused contagious diseases. These views were shared by Mizouri from Pavia, Valarianno Elbrero also from Pavia, and Elsiari from Milan.

It was not until the works and publications of Giocommo Elcermi in Milan and Agostino Bassi at Pavia University that the microbial origin of infectious diseases began to take shape. Their views and works were heavily influenced by the teachings of Francesco Redi and Spallanzani.[3]

Beginning as early as the 11th and 12th centuries, Italy gradually became a center for the development of philosophy, the arts, and a meteoric rise of trade with the rest of the world. In part, this was due to the fact that Italy, and more particularly Rome, became the center of Christendom. As early as 825 A.D. Pavia, which was the ancient capital of the Italian kingdom, boasted a university which over the years had included numerous scientific scholars.

In his excellent *History of the Italian People,* Giuliano Procacci details the influence that Italy had in commerce and in inviting pilgrims to Rome, thus contributing to the intellectual development of Italy. Procacci pointed out that the main pilgrim route to Rome entered the Po Valley by way of the Val d'Aosta, went through Pavia and on to Siena, Tuscany, and then Rome.

The improvements of the social standing of the people of Italy added profoundly in permitting an enlarged population to seek education. These attributes have been elaborated by Procacci in the comments of the German bishop Otto of Freising, who visited Italy:

The inhabitants of Italy still imitate the perspicacity of the ancient Romans in the ordering of towns and public matters. Indeed, they so much love liberty that to escape the arrogance of rulers they put themselves under the rule of consuls rather than of sovereigns. Since they know that there are three social classes among them: that is, the lords, the vavasours and the common people, to keep down pride they choose those consuls not from one but from each of the three social classes, and so that they shall not be carried away by the lust for power they change them almost year by year. So, since that land is almost entirely divided into cities, each of these cities has forced the inhabitants of the diocese to stay with her, and one may hardly find any noble or great man so powerful that he does not obey the rule of his city. And so as not to lack the means by which they can hold down their neighbours, they do not disdain to raise to knighthood and the honours of office young men of base birth, or any man practicing low manual work, whom other peoples keep as far as the plague from higher and freer activities: for this reason they greatly exceed the other cities of the world in wealth and power.

NOTES

1. The original volume written by Mondino rests in the library to this day at the University of Bologna. In August of 1988, on the occasion of the 9th Centennial representing the founding of the University of Bologna, Mondino's treatise was reprinted and made available to scholars. See the Appendix where reproductions from Mondino's seminal monograph are reproduced.

2. This factor of microorganisms causing fermentation being related to organisms that could cause infectious disease as concluded by Van Leeuwenhoek prompted Pasteur to essentially draw the same conclusion following his studies of fermentation.

3. An excellent chronological discourse on the early studies of investigators, principally Italians, that related infections of animals to an organism is contained in the volume by Carlo Francesco Cogrossi published in 1714, and this monograph was republished by the Italian Society for Microbiology on the occasion of the 6th International Congress of Microbiology held in Rome in 1953.

Chapter Two

Francesco Redi

Despite the frequent musings that diseases could be caused by invisible organisms, scholars still lacked technical evidence for their claims. Therefore, when infectious epidemics inundated a country, it provided an excellent opportunity for people to blame their political adversaries for the diseases. In some cases, innocent people were charged with the responsibility of causing such epidemics and were oftentimes killed in the streets by angry mobs.

The cholera epidemics, which were believed to have started in Africa and Asia in 1817, began to invade Russia and then Hungary and Germany. By 1835 the epidemic of cholera in many of the Italian states had reached such proportions that there were constant outbreaks of civil disobedience as a rebellion against political forces that were blamed for the very large number of deaths. Thus, epidemics that laid waste to Milan, Brescia, and other provinces of Italy—especially those that were under the domination of Austria—left about 22,000 dead out of approximately 43,000 cases of cholera. In the province of Lombardi, within a few months in 1836, about 32,000 people died out of approximately 60,000 that had been infected with cholera.

In order to understand the gradual transformation from the role of natural philosophers to investigations of the natural sciences that could properly be characterized as "research," it is necessary to understand the role of the institutions of education, especially during the period from the 16th to the beginning of the 18th century. The Italian system of education was essentially based on autonomous bodies called "colleges," which were actually self-governing trade guilds. Until approximately the middle of the 18th century, orders such as those of the Jesuits had acquired a monopoly over the teaching of courses such as mathematics and general physics. These faculties, unlike the institutes of higher education, were not subject to supervision by the secular governments, but received their authority only from the central authorities of the Roman curia and essentially the pope himself. At the University of Pavia, for example, professorships in the philosophical and theological disciplines were relegated to religious monasteries.

These colleges or guilds were essentially restricted to what can be characterized as gentile members of the community, and oftentimes there were rather rigid restrictions with regard to the geographical areas from which the students could be accepted and where they could practice.

The colleges not only had the absolute rights of admitting or rejecting applicants to these universities, but they could enact statutes that would give them the right to fine, suspend, and/or expel those that might be practicing without a license—regulations set down by the clergy.

The criteria as to the nobility of the family from which a student could be accepted to these colleges oftentimes demanded that at least two or three generations of the family had to be free of taint and of having labored in the trades.

Physicians were restricted to the treating of certain diseases and were barred from any intervention of the body by cutting or surgical procedure. Patients that had wounds or abscesses requiring surgical treatment were relegated to the barber-surgeons. The colleges of physicians enjoyed a monopoly of those that went to the university. They characterized as charlatans those that would seek to practice medicine outside of the university or guild system, including those who might have been rejected, not on the basis of their education or merit, but on the grounds of their birth and social standing.

Many cities and states, especially towards the end of the 17th century, had the prerogative to hire physicians and surgeons and contract with them to provide free health service for their citizens. Thus, a sort of faculty developed who were able to find employment outside the restrictive criteria for entrance into the colleges of physicians, gradually diminishing the power of the colleges.

The hospitals were almost entirely supervised and run by the church. Canon law exempted them from any supervision or inspection with regard to criteria of station, and they were able to train their own barber-surgeons and apothecaries. The hospital physicians and surgeons received a certificate, which essentially was a license to practice in the hospitals of the cities. This alternative to the restricted colleges overcame the bias of social standing as a criterion for entrance to the medical schools.

The idea that the state of health for any resulting pathology was the result of an imbalance of chemical substances in the body was maintained as a dogmatic explanation of disease of humans even as late as 1850. Consequently, those investigators that began to believe that small animals, parasites, and even living organisms that they could not see might be responsible for disease were ridiculed and challenged by the establishment. Even the distinguished

German chemist Justace von Liebig still retained the idea that disease was caused by a chemical imbalance of the body.

In order to possibly correct this imbalance, physicians introduced various procedures which included the use of leeches, cupping, bleeding, enemas, purgatives, and even sneezing powders. Cupping was achieved by utilizing a small glass cup approximately one and a half inches long by about 1 inch in diameter into which was placed a lit wafer. The wafer would burn up the oxygen and form a partial vacuum so that when the cup was placed over the skin of a patient, that part of the skin was sucked into the cup. This treatment, it was believed, relieved fevers and harmful substances that caused the disease which would be so eliminated from the body. Even as late as the early part of the 20th century, many barbershops still retained signs in their window indicating "We do Cupping."

Up to the beginning of the 18th century, the prevailing doctrine explaining the origin of many organisms was the concept of spontaneous generation; that live organisms could originate directly from non-living matter. The idea of spontaneous generation had its principal supporters during the early Egyptian periods, when it was claimed that beetles, which were originally not found in animal dung, could spontaneously arise from the dung.

The concept of spontaneous generation was accepted dogma both among the clergy and the scientific community. One of the first to undertake experiments to repudiate the concept of spontaneous generation was Francesco Redi, as seen in Figure 2.1. His father was a physician who worked for the grand duke of Tuscany, so Redi was destined for a good education. Redi attended the Jesuit schools in Florence.

Redi went to Florence to study such languages as French, German, and English and to attend the court of the Medici there. He became a member of the famous "Crusca Academy." He further became a member of the Academy of the Arcadia, where he began to develop the talent for conducting research. He ultimately became both a well-known scientific investigator and a proficient medical doctor. His scientific experiments were quoted in many treatises. Among them was the famous one, "Some Observations of Vipers," as shown in Figure 2.2. In this experiment, he may well have risked his own life by demonstrating that drinking the viper poison did not kill a person, but if injected into the blood could be fatal.

One of the most telling experiments of Redi was his demonstration of the lack of credibility of the theory of spontaneous generation.

In 1647, at the age of 20, he graduated from the University of Pisa with degrees in philosophy and medicine.

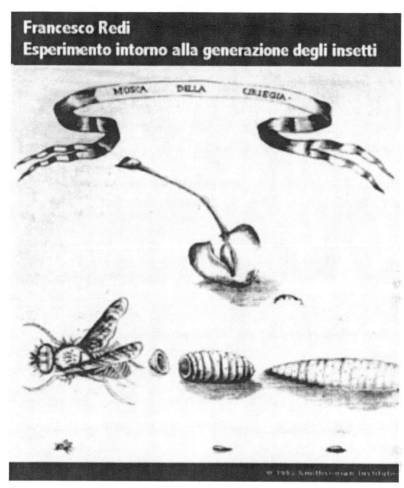

Francesco Redi
Esperimento intorno alla generazione degli insetti

Figure 2.1.   Francesco Redi debunks spontaneous generation.

Redi published a book entitled *The Experiences about the Generation of the Bugs.* He wrote:

I put in four flasks with wide mouths one sneak, some fish of river, four small eels of Arno River and a piece of calf and I locked very well the mouths of the flasks with paper and string. Afterward I placed in other four flasks the same things and left the mouths of flasks open. A short time later the meat and the fishes inside the open flasks became verminous, and after three weeks I saw many flies around flasks, but in the locked ones I've never seen a worm.

Some Observations of Vipers.

A curious *Italian*, called *Francesco Redi*, having lately had an opportunity, by the great number of Vipers, brought to the *Grand Luke* of *Tuscany* for the composing of *Theriac* or *Treacle*, to examine what is vulgarly delivered and believed concerning the Poyson of those Creatures, hath, (according to the account, given of it in the French *Journal des Scavans*, printed *January* 4. 166$\frac{2}{3}$) performed his undertaking with much exactness, and publish'd in an Italian tract, not yet come into *England*, these Observations.

1. He hath observed, that the poyson of Vipers is neither in their *Teeth*, nor in their *Tayle*, nor in their *Gall*; but in the two *Vesicles* or *Bladders*, which cover their teeth, and which coming to be compressed, when the Vipers bite, do emit a certain yellowish Liquor, that runs along the teeth and poysons the wound. Whereof he gives this proof, that he hath rub'd the wounds of many Animals with the *Gall* of Vipers, and pricked them with their *Teeth*, and yet no considerable ill accident follow'd upon it, but that as often as he rubbed the wounds with the said yellow Liquor, not one of them escaped.

2 Whereas commonly it hath hitherto been believed, that the poyson of Vipers being swallowed, was present death; this *Author*, after many reiterated Experiments, is said to have observed, that in Vipers there is neither Humour, nor Excrement, nor any part, not the *Gall* it self, that, being taken into the Body, kills. And he assures, that he hath seen men eat, and hath often made Bruit Animals swallow all that is esteem'd most poysonous in a Viper, yet without the least mischief to them.

Figure 2.2. Francesco Redi's experiment with viper poison.

To overcome his doubts that the lack of air circulating in the closed bottles would explain the results, he repeated the experiments using a gauze to cover the bottle opening and placed the gauze-covered bottle in a cage also covered with gauze. However, the results were exactly the same as in the first experiment. Despite the fact that Redi utilized the concept of a controlled experiment and despite the observations he made and reported, he was still convinced that some organisms could be generated spontaneously from dead matter.

One of the early investigators of the role of microorganisms in disease was Lazzaro Spallanzani. Redi's observations (1668 and 1684) were subsequently taken up and further developed by Spallanzani, whose distinguished career of highly diverse investigations left us with the legacy of this most versatile individual.

Redi died suddenly in his sleep in Pisa on March 1, 1697.

Chapter Three

Lazzaro Spallanzani

If I set out to prove something, I am no real scientist—I have to learn to follow where the facts lead me—I have to learn to whip my prejudices.

—Lazzaro Spallanzani

Spallanzani's father was a well-known attorney who lived in Scandiano, a town northeast of the Apennine Mountains. Spallanzani entered a Jesuit college at Reggio Emilia at the age of fifteen years. At the age of twenty, he went to the famous university at Bologna to study law. After three years of law study, Spallanzani decided that he preferred the natural sciences. At the age of twenty-four, he received a degree as a doctor of philosophy, and four years later he was ordained a priest.

In 1755, at the age of 26, Spallanzani began to teach logic, metaphysics, and the Greek language at a college in Reggio, Lombardy. Two years later, he was appointed a lecturer in mathematics at the University of Reggio Emilia; and in the following year, he was a professor of both Greek and French at another college.

Beginning in the summer of 1761, Spallanzani undertook a series of trips and investigations frequently in the Apennines and on occasion into Sicily and other parts of southern Italy. He wanted to observe and study the nature of the disposition of natural springs and the strata of these areas, including observations of many of the natural fauna and flora. His investigations were so productive that a report of his voyages was published in Pavia in six volumes. Many of these were translated into French, German, and English.

Spallanzani met the French naturalist Georges-Louis Leclerc, Comte de Buffon, and John Needham, a famous English priest and microscopist, in 1761. Buffon and Needham believed that all living things contain so-called "vital atoms" that are responsible for all the physiological activities of the body. They had postulated a theory that after death, these vital atoms would escape into the soil and be taken up by plants. The plants, in turn, would be introduced into animals and humans when soil products and plants were absorbed or taken intact as foods. Buffon and Needham also felt that minute organisms could be observed floating in water infusions of plant and animal tissue if the tissue was left to stand for extended periods of time. They, therefore, postulated that these are the "vital atoms" that had escaped from the organic material, which had been used to make the infusions.

Spallanzani took up the challenge and was influential in refuting this theory by his very well-controlled experiments, which became one of his greatest and most brilliant contributions. By 1767 Spallanzani, at the age of 38, had undertaken experiments to negate the concept of spontaneous generation.

Spallanzani was one of the first to begin to conduct what we might characterize as "controlled experiments." Although he voiced the idea that spontaneous generation could not occur, he was reluctant to abandon the concept completely. He was quoted as saying that there might be some special cases of spontaneous generation to explain findings which did not show the presence of living organisms. Obviously, at the time of Spallanzani, the presence of viruses had not yet been discovered. Otherwise, viruses could have explained disease states from which no organisms could be seen with the microscopes available at that time.

Spallanzani's studies concerning regeneration of lower animals and the results of his transplantation experiments were able to successfully demonstrate that the lower an animal is biologically, the greater regenerative power that animal will have. He also found that young of any given species have a greater capability of regenerating tissues than adults of the same species. Spallanzani was able to successfully transplant the head of one snail onto the body of another; these studies were published in 1768.

Spallanzani also investigated the role of semen in affecting the onset of the development of an egg, which ultimately results in the maturation of the egg into a living animal. The church-accepted, as well as scientifically accepted, dogma at that time was that all living things were created by God in the beginning, and that God encapsulated the germ for life within the female of each species. Thus, the developing embryo present in an egg was the result of the growth of this first germ that had been laid down by God at the creation, and such germs were transmitted from one generation to the next. Spallanzani was able to show that it required actual contact between an egg and semen for the development of an animal. By filtering semen through a porous paper, he observed that the more complete the filtration, the less effective the semen was in fertilizing an egg which developed into a living animal. Further, Spallanzani was also able to demonstrate that the bulk of the semen that was left behind on the paper frequently resulted in the development of a mature animal from the egg. Following such experiments, Spallanzani was probably the first person to artificially inseminate the eggs of lower animals and dogs.

Nevertheless, despite these observations by Spallanzani, he never overcame the accepted view at the time that the spermatozoa that could readily be seen in semen with a microscope were merely parasites and played no role in the activation of the germ plasma in an egg for the development of a living animal. In addition, Spallanzani never overcame the view that even his experiments, as well conducted as they were at the time, did not conclusively prove that spontaneous generation was not a viable concept.

Spallanzani, because of the prestige a chair at Pavia would offer, accepted a position at the University of Pavia, where he was appointed professor of natural history in 1769.

The University of Pavia is one of the oldest universities in Europe. A higher institute of education was established in Pavia in 825 A.D. by King Lotarius. The institute was primarily devoted to the teaching of ecclesiastical and civil law. The university was enlarged and ultimately established as a major university by Emperor Charles IV in 1361.

Spallanzani's lectures frequently repeated the seminal experiments that he had performed in 1767 in order to put to rest the concept of spontaneous generation as shown in Figure 3.1.

It is 2:30 in the afternoon at the University of Pavia. Twenty-seven young men have registered to take a course in natural history under the tutelage of Lazzaro Spallanzani, professor of natural history and an ordained priest. Spallanzani begins:

This morning I have taken a piece of meat and cut it into small pieces. I have added the meat to two gallons of water contained in a pot, added a few drams of sugar and salt. I proceeded to boil this broth for approximately two to three hours. I then poured the broth through six layers of cloth to remove all of the solids, leaving a nice clear broth liquid that you see before you. I will now add an equal amount of this broth to four flasks of similar size. Flask number one, I shall leave open on this table. Flask number two, I shall apply a cork so sealing the contents and protecting it further from air. Flask number three and flask number four, I will place over this fire, and permit the contents of the flasks to reach a boil. We will now boil the contents of flasks three and four for one hour. At the end of the hour, I shall place a cork and seal flask number four. Flask number three will be left exposed to air. All four flasks will be left on this desk until tomorrow at 10 A.M., when we shall reconvene.

Spallanzani's Experiment

What causes microbes to form in
decaying broth?
Hypothesis: Microbes come from the air.
Boiling will kill microorganisms.
Spallanzani put broth into four flasks

> This outline with drawings
> depicting Spallanzani's experiment
> is reproduced here with permission
> from the Kent School District in
> Kent, Washington.

     Flask 1 as left open.
     Flask 2 was sealed.
     Flask 3 was boiled and then left open.
     Flask 4 was boiled and then sealed.

Spallanzani's Experiment – Step 1

Flask 1

     Left Open
     Turned cloudy
     Microbes were found

Spallanzani's Experiment – Step 2

Flask 2

     Sealed
     Turned cloudy
     Microbes were found

Spallanzani's Experiment – Step 3

Flask 3

     Boiled and left open
     Turned cloudy
     Microbes were found

Spallanzani's Experiment – Step 4

Flask 4

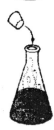

     Boiled and sealed
     Did not turn cloudy
     Microbes not found

Figure 3.1. Spallanzani's experiments in killing bacteria.

The next morning the students convened and Spallanzani begins:

> Notice that the first three flasks all have become very cloudy, but that flask number four still retains a clear broth exactly as we placed it into the flask and boiled it. We are obliged to conclude that boiling, as is well known, can destroy life, but we must accept the fact that very small living animals are present in the air around us that we cannot see with our eyes, and as long as the flask is left open, despite being boiled—the same as flask number four—these minute living animals will get into the flask and begin to grow and multiply. Flask number four was sealed immediately after being boiled, and therefore nothing living from the air could get into the flask and grow. If spontaneous generation were a characteristic that would explain the origin of living things from non-living things, then we would have expected flask number four to show the same over-growth and cloudiness that we find in the other three flasks.

Spallanzani asks, "Are there any questions?"

A student responds, "Can the results be explained by someone coming into the room during the night and deliberately adding some nutritive factor that caused flasks one, two, and three to become very cloudy and presumably overgrown?"

Spallanzani was quick to reply: "I suppose it is possible, but since anyone of you can easily repeat exactly the experiment I have demonstrated and can perform this experiment for themselves, this will ensure that your suggestion of someone tampering with the flask would not have occurred."

Spallanzani queried again, "Any other questions?"

A student responded: "Can we not explain that the exposure to air regard-less of whether the broth was boiled or not resulted in a reaction between those components of air and the broth to cause the cloudiness that we see in flasks one, two, and three, whereas, placing the cork in flask number four prevented such a reaction from the air?"

Spallanzani answered, "Perhaps, that might be considered, but the flasks were never full. Even in flask number four, placing the cork in the neck of the flask after it was boiled left plenty of air in the flask, if in fact, the air in the flask was responsible for causing the cloudiness in the broth."

"Ah," quickly answered a curious student, "but when the flask is boiled, the boiling represents the change in state from a liquid to a gaseous state, and the air is expelled together with the gaseous broth during the boiling."

Spallanzani replied:

> Well, I think we can answer and satisfy your doubts by taking a small amount of each of the broths in flasks one, two, three, and four, placing a drop on a small slide and examining the contents of the slide under this microscope. I want you to come up and look through the microscope and see what is present in the broths of flasks one, two, and three that is completely absent from flask number four.

The first students came up and looked through the microscope after the slides had been prepared and placed under the lens of the microscope. They saw what they believed to be small little animals swimming around in the broth from flasks one, two, and three, but they saw nothing moving in the broth from flask number four. When the students had satisfied themselves that nothing was moving and therefore nothing was living in flask number four, Spallanzani went on to point out that this experiment provided the controls considering and proving that air contains living organisms that are so small that we cannot see them except under a microscope, and that boiling would kill these organisms.

He indicated, "However, we can conceive that under certain conditions, spontaneous generation may well occur, but in most cases as we have demonstrated, it cannot be that living organisms will arise from dead inanimate matter such as broth."

The rather crude but opportune development of a medium by Spallanzani for growing microorganisms made it possible for the first time to grow bacteria in large numbers. Small pieces of meat, sugar, and salt boiled for a few hours in water would provide a very nutritious medium for many pathogenic organisms. Because this medium could be sterilized by boiling, it would be possible to determine those conditions that would destroy living organisms and prevent their multiplication. The seminal series of experiments by Spallanzani were later repeated by other investigators who followed essentially the same procedures.

By observing the growth of bacteria in the nutrient broths he prepared, Spallanzani was able to conclude that bacteria can multiply by dividing into two. These "daughter" microorganisms can ultimately divide again into two, and such a division can proceed as a geometric progression which can readily explain why the culture medium would become overgrown in a relatively short period of time. Spallanzani became the first person to clearly point out that the multiplication of bacteria by such a geometric progression can reach enormous numbers of organisms in a relatively short time. He also was first to explain why such numbers can overcome defense mechanisms of the body in either man or animals and result in a sufficient pathology to cause disease and ultimately death.

In order for his students to understand this capability, he provided the following example:

In order for you to understand the enormity of the capability of bacteria to multiply geometrically, let me give you the following example: You have an uncle that is in the business of selling goods and you want experience for a month in order to learn his trade, so you go to him and you say, "Uncle, I just want to work for you for experience, but as a token gesture, pay me a penny the first day, two cents the second day, four cents the next day, eight cents the next day, etc., doubling this sum until at the end of a 30-day month, I shall have learned my trade and you shall pay me those relatively few pennies that have accumulated in the course of a month." Now then tell me how much money your uncle would owe you at the end of 30 days.

One student offered that starting with one penny, if one were to take one penny to the 30th power, representing the 30 days in the month it would give us the correct answer as to how many pennies we would be owed.

Spallanzani replied:

No, no, no, one penny to any power—to a power of 10, 100, or 1,000 is still one. You have to multiply by two the amount from the previous day to the next day until you have done this 30 times. The answer is 396,361,728. If you started therefore, with one bacterium, as I have discovered that many of these bacteria can multiply once every 30 minutes, then you would not have to wait an entire month in order to get that many bacteria into the body. Who is going to calculate for me how long it would take to reach 396,361,728 bacteria if they multiplied once every 30 minutes and they multiplied as a geometric progression assuming that there was enough good food for all of them to keep on growing?

Spallanzani conducted controlled experiments in which he was able to demonstrate that microorganisms would grow on a nutrient medium, such as gravy. However, if the gravy was boiled and the boiled gravy was prevented from being exposed to air, no microorganisms developed. He used these experiments to refute the theory of spontaneous generation; although he was not willing to completely capitulate to the idea that spontaneous generation could not occur under certain circumstances.

By these relatively simple controlled series of experiments and other brilliant experiments that he made throughout his career, Spallanzani paved the way for those who followed him in studying the role of microorganisms as a cause of disease.

Spallanzani (1766, 1767(a), 1767(b), and 1773) spent the rest of his life in highly divergent studies of biology, plant life, and mineral structure. He also conducted experiments on the circulation of blood and was able to show that the pumping of the heart was transmitted throughout the entire arterial system. His collection of fossils and biological specimens significantly enlarged the Museum of Natural History at the University of Pavia and became one of the most magnificent collections in Italy.

Spallanzani's courses in natural history were very well attended. It was at Pavia under the influence of Spallanzani that a student named Agostino Bassi came to veer his interest in law in order to pursue courses in the natural sciences.

Spallanzani died on February 11, 1799.

Chapter Four

Edward Jenner and the Concept of Vaccination

Contemporaneously with Spallanzani, an English country doctor by the name of Edward Jenner was intrigued by observations he had been making for a number of years—that there might be a relationship between the occurrence of smallpox in humans and cowpox and swinepox.

Edward Jenner was born in the small English town of Berkeley, in Gloucestershire. By the time he was 5 years old, both of his parents had died and he was put into the care of his eldest sister. Jenner, himself, while attending school as a young boy, was inoculated against smallpox by following a practice which had originated in China. The practice involved taking a small amount of the pox exudate from a lesion of a patient who had smallpox and inoculating such exudate into the skin of a healthy person. It presumably was intended to provide protection against the ultimate challenge of the smallpox organism.

At the age of 14, Jenner was apprenticed to Dr. Daniel Ludlow and was trained to become a surgeon. At the age of 23, he returned to the village of Berkeley and began his practice as the town doctor and surgeon.

Smallpox at the beginning of the 18th century and for some period thereafter was devastating the European countryside. Almost 33 percent of all people who contracted smallpox died, and most of the fatalities were young children or infants. Because smallpox was so widespread and the pox scars were so evident on the bodies of those that had recovered, one of the distinguishing characteristics on a wanted poster for a criminal in England at that time was that the criminal did not have a pox mark on his face.

Turkish physicians had been practicing the inoculation with smallpox by procuring a small amount of the pox exudate and injecting it into an individual who had never been exposed to smallpox. The idea that a number of repeated small inoculations of material that could cause disease might serve to protect against future exposure to that disease stemmed from observations, primarily in central Europe, where small amounts of arsenic could be taken and the dose increased over a period of time, ultimately rendering the person immune to a lethal dose of arsenic if swallowed. This observation, when extended to the treatment of infectious diseases, ultimately resulted in the practice of homeopathy in which the primary axiom was *Similia Similibus Curentur* (Like cures like).

In 1721, the wife of the British ambassador to the Orient, Lady Mary Montagu, began to promote the use of vaccination using a small amount of smallpox exudate as she had observed being practiced in China. Members of the Royal Family in England were so inoculated. However, utilizing the pus from a person infected with smallpox was not always protective against the disease and, in a number of cases, proved fatal to those thus inoculated. This was because there were no methods available to control the dosage that was inoculated, nor to avoid contamination.

The first recorded use of the cowpox virus (vaccinia) to inoculate someone as a protective measure against smallpox was documented in 1774, when an English farmer, Benjamin Jesty, was reputed to have inoculated his wife with the virus obtained from a farmer Elford of Chittenhall, near the village of Yetminster.

Jenner had heard what were characterized as "old wives' tales" that milkmaids could not get smallpox. If this were true, there might be a connection between the fact that milkmaids procured blister-type lesions on their hands when they milked cows, but did not get the smallpox infection itself. Jenner, therefore, felt that a non-lethal inoculation with cowpox might prevent the smallpox from resulting in a disease. In order to test this theory, Jenner found a milkmaid named Sarah Nelmes who had such cowpox lesions on her hands from milking a cow called "Blossom." The teats of the cow had in fact developed small blisters. On May 14, 1796, Jenner took some of the pus from the blisters on the hands of the milkmaid and injected it into a healthy 8-year-old boy named James Phipps. Over a period of a number of days, Jenner injected more of the pus into James Phipps, gradually increasing the dosage. After a series of increasing doses of injection, Jenner, in a most courageous leap of faith, injected Phipps with the actual pus from a smallpox lesion. The boy became ill, but after a short period of time he made a total recovery and did not show the scourge of a full-blown smallpox disease. Phipps was challenged with injections of pus from smallpox lesions for a number of years thereafter and remained immune to smallpox.

Jenner reported a series of experiments in order to demonstrate the protective effect of material taken from cowpox when a patient was ultimately challenged with smallpox. The following cases illustrate the experimental design and the confidence that Jenner had in indulging in such human experiments, especially with children including his own son. Excerpts from Jenner's own case histories are shown in Figure 4.1.

AN

INQUIRY

INTO

THE CAUSES AND EFFECTS

OF

THE VARIOLÆ VACCINÆ,

A DISEASE

DISCOVERED IN SOME OF THE WESTERN COUNTIES OF ENGLAND,

PARTICULARLY

GLOUCESTERSHIRE,

AND KNOWN BY THE NAME OF

THE COW POX.

BY EDWARD JENNER, M.D. F.R.S. &c.

——— QUID NOBIS CERTIUS IPSIS

SENSIBUS ESSE POTEST, QUO VERA AC FALSA NOTEMUS.

LUCRETIUS.

London:

PRINTED, FOR THE AUTHOR,

BY SAMPSON LOW, N.º 7, BERWICK STREET, SOHO:

AND SOLD BY LAW, AVE-MARIA LANE; AND MURRAY AND HIGHLEY, FLEET STREET

1798.

Figure 4.1.   Case histories for the smallpox vaccine of Edward Jenner.

TO

C. H PARRY, M. D.

AT BATH.

MY DEAR FRIEND,

IN the prefent age of fcientific inveftigation, it is remarkable that a difeafe of fo peculiar a nature as the Cow Pox, which has appeared in this and fome of the neighbouring counties for fuch a feries of years, fhould fo long have efcaped particular attention. Finding the prevailing notions on the fubject, both among men of our profeffion and others, extremely vague and indeterminate, and conceiving that facts might ap-

Figure 4.1. Continued.

[iv]

pear at once both curious and ufeful, I have infti-
tuted as ftrict an inquiry into the caufes and effects
of this fingular malady as local circumftances would
admit.

The following pages are the refult, which, from
motives of the moft affectionate regard, are dedi-
cated to you, by

Your fincere Friend,

EDWARD JENNER.

Berkeley, Gloucefterfhire,
 June 21ft, 1798.

Figure 4.1. Continued.

AN

INQUIRY,

&c. &c.

THE deviation of Man from the ſtate in which he was originally placed by Nature ſeems to have proved to him a prolific ſource of Diſeaſes. From the love of ſplendour, from the indulgences of luxury, and from his fondneſs for amuſement, he has familiariſed himſelf with a great number of animals, which may not originally have been intended for his aſſociates.

Figure 4.1. Continued.

[2]

The Wolf, difarmed of ferocity, is now pillowed in the lady's lap*. The Cat, the little Tyger of our ifland, whofe natural home is the foreft, is equally domefticated and careffed. The Cow, the Hog, the Sheep, and the Horfe, are all, for a variety of purpofes, brought under his care and dominion.

There is a difeafe to which the Horfe, from his ftate of domeftication, is frequently fubject. The Farriers have termed it *the Greafe*. It is an inflammation and fwelling in the heel, from which iffues matter poffeffing properties of a very peculiar kind, which feems capable of generating a difeafe in the Human Body (after it has undergone the modification which I fhall prefently fpeak of), which bears fo ftrong a refemblance to the Small Pox, that I think it highly probable it may be the fource of that difeafe.

* The late Mr. John Hunter proved, by experiments, that the Dog is the Wolf in a degenerated ftate.

Figure 4.1. Continued.

[3]

In this Dairy Country a great number of Cows are kept, and the office of milking is performed indifcriminately by Men and Maid Servants. One of the former having been appointed to apply dreffings to the heels of a Horfe affeéted with *the Greafe*, and not paying due attention to cleanli-nefs, incautioufly bears his part in milking the Cows, with fome particles of the infeétious matter ad-hering to his fingers. When this is the cafe, it commonly happens that a difeafe is communicated to the Cows, and from the Cows to the Dairy-maids, which fpreads through the farm until moft of the cattle and domeftics feel its unpleafant confe-quences. This difeafe has obtained the name of the Cow Pox. It appears on the nipples of the Cows in the form of irregular puftules. At their firft appearance they are commonly of a palifh blue, or rather of a colour fomewhat approaching to livid, and are furrounded by an eryfipelatous in-

Figure 4.1.   Continued.

[4]

flammation. Thefe puftules, unlefs a timely re-
medy be applied, frequently degenerate into phagedenic ulcers, which prove extremely troublefome   The animals become indifpofed, and the
fecretion of milk is much leffened. Inflamed fpots
now begin to appear on different parts of the hands
of the domeftics employed in milking, and fometimes on the wrifts, which quickly run on to fup-
puration, firft affuming the appearance of the fmall
vefications produced by a burn. Moft commonly
they appear about the joints of the fingers, and
at their extremities; but whatever parts are af-
ected, if the fituation will admit, thefe fuperficial
fuppurations put on a circular form, with their
edges more elevated than their centre, and of a

Figure 4.1. Continued.

[5]

colour diftantly approaching to blue. Abforption
takes place, and tumours appear in each axilla.
The fyftem becomes affected — the pulfe is quick-
ened; and fhiverings, with general laffitude and
pains about the loins and limbs, with vomiting,
come on. The head is painful, and the patient is
now and then even affected with delirium. Thefe
fymptoms, varying in their degrees of violence,
generally continue from one day to three or four,
leaving ulcerated fores about the hands, which, from
the fenfibility of the parts, are very troublefome,
and commonly heal flowly, frequently becoming
phagedenic, like thofe from whence they fprung.
The lips, noftrils, eyelids, and other parts of the
body, are fometimes affected with fores; but thefe
evidently arife from their being needlefsly rubbed
or fcratched with the patient's infected fingers.
No eruptions on the fkin have followed the decline
of the feverifh fymptoms in any inftance that has

Figure 4.1. Continued.

[6]

come under my infpe&ion, one only excepted, and in this cafe a very few appeared on the arms : they were very minute, of a vivid red colour, and foon died away without advancing to maturation ; fo that I cannot determine whether they had any conne&ion with the preceding fymptoms.

Thus the difeafe makes its progrefs from the Horfe to the nipple of the Cow, and from the Cow to the Human Subje&.

Morbid matter of various kinds, when abforbed into the fyftem, may produce effe&s in fome degree fimilar; but what renders the Cow-pox virus fo extremely fingular, is, that the perfon who has been thus affe&ed is for ever after fecure from the infec-tion of the Small Pox; neither expofure to the variolous effluvia, nor the infertion of the matter into the fkin, producing this diftemper.

Figure 4.1. Continued.

[11   ]

CASE II.

SARAH PORTLOCK, of this place, was infected with
the Cow Pox, when a Servant at a Farmer's in the neighbourhood, twenty-seven years ago*.

In the year 1792, conceiving herself, from this circum-
stance, secure from the infection of the Small Pox, she
nursed one of her own children who had accidentally
caught the disease, but no indisposition ensued.—During
the time she remained in the infected room, variolous
matter was inserted into both her arms, but without any
further effect than in the preceding case.

---

* I have purposely selected several cases in which the disease had appeared
at a very distant period previous to the experiments made with variolous
matter, to shew that the change produced in the constitution is not affected by
time.

Figure 4.1.   Continued.

[12]

CASE III.

JOHN PHILLIPS, a Tradefman of this town, had the Cow Pox at fo early a period as nine years of age. At the age of fixty-two I inoculated him, and was very careful in felecting matter in its moft active ftate. It was taken from the arm of a boy juft before the commencement of the eruptive fever, and inftantly inferted. It very fpeedily produced a fting-like feel in the part. An efflorefcence appeared, which on the fourth day was rather extenfive, and fome degree of pain and ftiffnefs were felt about the fhoulder; but on the fifth day thefe fymptoms began to difappear, and in a day or two after went entirely off, without producing any effect on the fyftem.

Figure 4.1. Continued.

[13]

CASE IV.

MARY BARGE, of Woodford, in this parifh, was inoculated with variolous matter in the year 1791. An efflorefcence of a palifh red colour foon appeared about the
parts where the matter was inferted, and fpread itfelf rather
extenfively, but died away in a few days without producing
any variolous fymptoms*. She has fince been repeatedly
employed as a nurfe to Small-pox patients, without expe-
riencing any ill confequences. This woman had the Cow
Pox when fhe lived in the fervice of a Farmer in this parifh
thirty-one years before.

---

  * It is remarkable that variolous matter, when the fyftem is difpofed to rejeft
it, fhould excite inflammation on the part to which it is applied more fpeedily
than when it produces the Small Pox. Indeed it becomes almoft a criterion by
which we can determine whether the infeftion will be received or not. It feems
as if a change, which endures through life, had been produced in the aftion, or
difpofition to aftion, in the veffels of the fkin; and it is remarkable too, that
whether this change has been effefted by the Small Pox, or the Cow Pox, that
the difpofition to fudden cuticular inflammation is the fame on the application of
variolous matter.

Figure 4.1. Continued.

[14]

CASE V.

MRS. H——, a refpectable Gentlewoman of this town, had the Cow Pox when very young. She received the infection in rather an uncommon manner: it was given by means of her handling fome of the fame utenfils * which were in ufe among the fervants of the family, who had the difeafe from milking infected cows. Her hands had many of the Cow-pox fores upon them, and they were communicated to her nofe, which became inflamed and very much fwoln. Soon after this event Mrs. H—— was expofed to the contagion of the Small Pox, where it was fcarcely poffible for her to have efcaped, had fhe been fufceptible of it, as fhe regularly attended a relative who had the difeafe in fo violent a degree that it proved fatal to him.

---

* When the Cow Pox has prevailed in the dairy, it has often been communicated to thofe who have not milked the cows, by the handle of the milk pail.

Figure 4.1. Continued.

[15]

In the year 1778 the Small Pox prevailed very much at
Berkeley, and Mrs. H—— not feeling perfectly satisfied
respecting her safety (no indisposition having followed her
exposure to the Small Pox) I inoculated her with active
variolous matter. The same appearance followed as in the
preceding cases — an efflorescence on the arm without any
effect on the constitution.

CASE VI.

IT is a fact so well known among our Dairy Farmers,
that those who have had the Small Pox either escape the
Cow Pox or are disposed to have it slightly; that as soon as
the complaint shews itself among the cattle, assistants are
procured, if possible, who are thus rendered less susceptible
of it, otherwise the business of the farm could scarcely go
forward.

In the month of May, 1796, the Cow Pox broke out at
Mr. Baker's, a Farmer who lives near this place. The

Figure 4.1. Continued.

[16]

difeafe was communicated by means of a cow which was purchafed in an infeɛted ftate at a neighbouring fair, and not one of the Farmer's cows (confifting of thirty) which were at that time milked efcaped the contagion. The family confifted of a man fervant, two dairymaids, and a fervant boy, who, with the Farmer himfelf, were twice a day employed in milking the cattle. The whole of this family, except Sarah Wynne, one of the dairymaids, had gone through the Small Pox. The confequence was, that the Farmer and the fervant boy efcaped the infeɛtion of the Cow Pox entirely, and the fervant man and one of the maid fervants had each of them nothing more than a fore on one of their fingers, which produced no diforder in the fyftem. But the other dairymaid, Sarah Wynne, who never had the Small Pox, did not efcape in fo eafy a manner. She caught the complaint from the cows, and was affeɛted with the fymptoms defcribed in the 5th page in fo violent a degree, that fhe was confined to her bed, and rendered incapable for feveral days of purfuing her ordinary vocations in the farm.

Figure 4.1. Continued.

[17]

March 28th, 1797, I inoculated this girl, and carefully rubbed the variolous matter into two flight incifions made upon the left arm. A little inflammation appeared in the ufual manner around the parts where the matter was inferted, but fo early as the fifth day it vanifhed entirely without producing any effect on the fyftem.

CASE VII.

ALTHOUGH the preceding hiftory pretty clearly evinces that the conftitution is far lefs fufceptible of the contagion of the Cow Pox after it has felt that of the Small Pox, and although in general, as I have obferved, they who have had the Small Pox, and are employed in milking cows which are infected with the Cow Pox, either efcape the diforder, or have fores on the hands without feeling any general indifpofition, yet the animal economy is fubject to fome variation in this refpect, which the following relation will point out:

Figure 4.1. Continued.

[18]

In the fummer of the year 1796 the Cow Pox appeared at the Farm of Mr. Andrews, a confiderable dairy adjoining to the town of Berkeley. It was communicated, as in the preceding inftance, by an infected cow purchafed at a fair in the neighbourhood. The family confifted of the Farmer, his wife, two fons, a man and a maid fervant; all of whom, except the Farmer (who was fearful of the confequences), bore a part in milking the cows. The whole of them, ex-clufive of the man fervant, had regularly gone through the Small Pox; but in this cafe no one who milked the cows efcaped the contagion. All of them had fores upon their hands, and fome degree of general indifpofition, preceded by pains and tumours in the axillæ: but there was no com-parifon in the feverity of the difeafe as it was felt by the fervant man, who had efcaped the Small Pox, and by thofe of the family who had not, for, while he was confined to his bed, they were able, without much inconvenience, to follow their ordinary bufinefs.

Figure 4.1. Continued.

[19]

February the 13th, 1797, I availed myfelf of an opportunity of inoculating William Rodway, the fervant man above alluded to. Variolous matter was inferted into both his arms; in the right by means of fuperficial incifions, and into the left by flight punctures into the cutis. Both were perceptibly inflamed on the third day. After this the inflammation about the punctures foon died away, but a fmall appearance of eryfipelas was manifeft about the edges of the incifions till the eighth day, when a little uneafinefs was felt for the fpace of half an hour in the right axilla. The inflammation then haftily difappeared without producing the moft diftant mark of affection of the fyftem.

Figure 4.1. Continued.

[20]

CASE VIII.

ELIZABETH WYNNE, aged fifty-feven, lived as a
fervant with a neighbouring Farmer thirty-eight years ago.
She was then a dairymaid, and the Cow Pox broke out
among the cows. She caught the difeafe with the reft of
the family, but, compared with them, had it in a very
flight degree, one very fmall fore only breaking out on the
little finger of her left hand, and fcarcely any perceptible
indifpofition following it.

As the malady had fhewn itfelf in fo flight a manner,
and as it had taken place at fo diftant a period of her life, I
was happy with the opportunity of trying the effects of
variolous matter upon her conftitution, and on the 28th of
March, 1797, I inoculated her by making two fuperficial
incifions on the left arm, on which the matter was cautioufly
rubbed. A little efflorefcence foon appeared, and a tin-

Figure 4.1. Continued.

[21]

gling fenfation was felt about the parts where the matter was inferted until the third day, when both began to fubfide. and fo early as the fifth day it was evident that no indifpofition would follow.

CASE IX.

ALTHOUGH the Cow Pox fhields the conftitution from the Small Pox, and the Small Pox proves a protection againft its own future poifon, yet it appears that the human body is again and again fufceptible of the infectious matter of the Cow Pox, as the following hiftory will demonftrate:

William Smith, of Pyrton in this parifh, contracted this difeafe when he lived with a neighbouring Farmer in the year 1780. One of the horfes belonging to the farm had fore heels, and it fell to his lot to attend him. By thefe means the infection was carried to the cows, and from the cows it was communicated to Smith. On one of his hands

Figure 4.1. Continued.

[22]

were feveral ulcerated fores, and he was affected with fuch fymptoms as have been before defcribed.

In the year 1791 the Cow Pox broke out at another farm where he then lived as a fervant, and he became affected with it a fecond time; and in the year 1794 he was fo unfortunate as to catch it again. The difeafe was equally as fevere the fecond and third time as it was on the firft *.

In the fpring of the year 1795 he was twice inoculated, but no affection of the fyftem could be produced from the variolous matter; and he has fince affociated with thofe who had the Small Pox in its moft contagious ftate without feeling any effect from it.

* This is not the cafe in general — a fecond attack is commonly very flight, and fo, I am informed, it is among the cows.

Figure 4.1. Continued.

[23]

CASE X.

SIMON NICHOLS lived as a fervant with Mr. Brom-edge, a gentleman who refides on his own farm in this parifh, in the year 1782. He was employed in applying dreffings to the fore heels of one of his mafter's horfes, and at the fame time affifted in milking the cows. The cows became affected in confequence, but the difeafe did not fhew itfelf on their nipples till feveral weeks after he had begun to drefs the horfe. He quitted Mr. Bromedge's fervice, and went to another farm without any fores upon him; but here his hands foon began to be affected in the common way, and he was much indifpofed with the ufual fymptoms. Concealing the nature of the malady from Mr. Cole, his new mafter, and being there alfo employed in milking, the Cow Pox was communicated to the cows.

Figure 4.1.   Continued.

[24]

Some years afterwards Nichols was employed in a farm where the Small Pox broke out, when I inoculated him with feveral other patients, with whom he continued during the whole time of their confinement. His arm inflamed, but neither the inflammation nor his affociating with the inoculated family produced the leaft effect upon his conftitution.

CASE XI.

WILLIAM STINCHCOMB was a fellow fervant with Nichols at Mr. Bromedge's Farm at the time the cattle had the Cow Pox, and he was unfortunately infected by them. His left hand was very feverely affected with feveral corroding ulcers, and a tumour of confiderable fize appeared in the axilla of that fide. His right hand had only one fmall fore upon it, and no fore difcovered itfelf in the corresponding axilla.

Figure 4.1. Continued.

[25   ]

In the year 1792 Stinchcomb was inoculated with variolous matter, but no confequences enfued beyond a little
inflammation in the arm for a few days. A large party
were inoculated at the fame time, fome of whom had the
difeafe in a more violent degree than is commonly feen
from inoculation. He purpofely affociated with them, but
could not receive the Small Pox.

During the fickening of fome of his companions, their
fymptoms fo ftrongly recalled to his mind his own ftate
when fickening with the Cow Pox, that he very pertinently
remarked their ftriking fimilarity.

Figure 4.1.   Continued.

[26]

CASE XII.

THE Paupers of the village of Tortworth, in this county, were inoculated by Mr. Henry Jenner, Surgeon, of Berkeley, in the year 1795. Among them, eight patients prefented themfelves who had at different periods of their lives had the Cow Pox. One of them, Hefter Walkley, I attended with that difeafe when fhe lived in the fervice of a Farmer in the fame village in the year 1782; but neither this woman, nor any other of the patients who had gone through the Cow Pox, received the variolous infection either from the arm or from mixing in the fociety of the other patients who were inoculated at the fame time. This ftate of fecurity proved a fortunate circumftance, as many of the poor women were at the fame time in a ftate of pregnancy.

Figure 4.1. Continued.

[27]

CASE XIII.

One inſtance has occurred to me of the fyſtem being affected from the matter iſſuing from the heels of horſes, and of its remaining afterwards unſuſceptible of the variolous contagion; another, where the Small Pox appeared obſcurely; and a third, in which its complete exiſtence was poſitively aſcertained.

Firſt, THOMAS PEARCE, is the ſon of a Smith and Farrier near to this place. He never had the Cow Pox; but, in conſequence of dreſſing horſes with ſore heels at his father's, when a lad, he had ſores on his fingers which ſuppurated, and which occaſioned a pretty ſevere indiſpoſition. Six years afterwards I inſerted variolous matter into his arm repeatedly, without being able to produce any thing more than ſlight inflammation, which appeared very ſoon

Figure 4.1.   Continued.

[28]

after the matter was applied, and afterwards I expofed him to the contagion of the Small Pox with as little effect *.

CASE XIV.

Secondly, Mr. JAMES COLE, a Farmer in this parifh, had a difeafe from the fame fource as related in the preceding cafe, and fome years after was inoculated with variolous matter. He had a little pain in the axilla, and felt a flight indifpofition for three or four hours. A few eruptions fhewed themfelves on the forehead, but they very foon difappeared without advancing to maturation.

---

* It is a remarkable fact, and well known to many, that we are frequently foiled in our endeavours to communicate the Small Pox by inoculation to blackfmiths, who in the country are farriers. They often, as in the above inftance, either refift the contagion entirely, or have the difeafe anomaloufly. Shall we not be able now to account for this on a rational principle ?

Figure 4.1. Continued.

[29]

CASE XV.

Although in the two former inftances the fyftem feemed to be fecured, or nearly fo, from variolous infection, by the abforption of matter from fores produced by the difeafed heels of horfes, yet the following cafe decifively proves that this cannot be entirely relied upon, until a difeafe has been generated by the morbid matter from the horfe on the nipple of the cow, and paffed through that medium to the human fubject.

Mr. ABRAHAM RIDDIFORD, a Farmer at Stone in this parifh, in confequence of dreffing a mare that had fore heels, was affected with very painful fores in both his hands, tumours in each axilla, and fevere and general indifpofition. A Surgeon in the neighbourhood attended him, who, knowing the fimilarity between the appearance of the fores upon his hands and thofe produced by the

Figure 4.1. Continued.

[30]

Cow Pox, and being acquainted alfo with the effects of that difeafe on the human conftitution, affured him that he never need to fear the infection of the Small Pox; but this affertion proved fallacious, for, on being expofed to the infection upwards of twenty years afterwards, he caught the difeafe, which took its regular courfe in a very mild way. There certainly was a difference perceptible, although it is not eafy to defcribe it, in the general appearance of the puftules from that which we commonly fee. Other practitioners, who vifited the patient at my requeft, agreed with me in this point, though there was no room left for fufpicion as to the reality of the difeafe, as I inoculated fome of his family from the puftules, who had the Small Pox, with its ufual appearances, in confequence.

Figure 4.1. Continued.

[3¹]

CASE XVI.

SARAH NELMES, a dairymaid at a Farmer's near this place, was infected with the Cow Pox from her mafter's cows in May, 1796. She received the infection on a part of the hand which had been previoufly in a flight degree injured by a fcratch from a thorn. A large puftulous fore and the ufual fymptoms accompanying the difeafe were produced in confequence. The puftule was fo expreffive of the true character of the Cow Pox, as it commonly appears upon the hand, that I have given a reprefentation of it in the annexed plate. The two fmall puftules on the wrifts arofe alfo from the application of the virus to fome minute abrafions of the cuticle, but the livid tint, if they ever had any, was not confpicuous at the time I faw the patient. The puftule on the fore finger fhews the difeafe in an earlier ftage. It did not actually appear on the hand of

Figure 4.1. Continued.

[32]

this young woman, but was taken from that of another, and is annexed for the purpofe of reprefenting the malady after it has newly appeared.

CASE XVII.

THE more accurately to obferve the progrefs of the infection, I felected a healthy boy, about eight years old, for the purpofe of inoculation for the Cow Pox. The matter was taken from a fore on the hand of a dairymaid *, who was infected by her mafter's cows, and it was inferted, on the 14th of May, 1796, into the arm of the boy by means of two fuperficial incifions, barely penetrating the cutis, each about half an inch long.

* From the fore on the hand of Sarah Nelmes. — See the preceding cafe and the plate.

Figure 4.1. Continued.

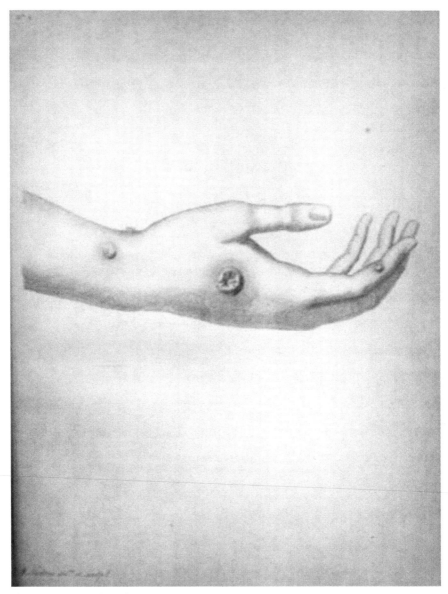

Figure 4.1.   Continued.

[33]

On the feventh day he complained of uneafinefs in the axilla, and on the ninth he became a little chilly, loft his appetite, and had a flight head-ach. During the whole of this day he was perceptibly indifpofed, and fpent the night with fome degree of reftleffnefs, but on the day following he was perfectly well.

The appearance of the incifions in their progrefs to a ftate of maturation were much the fame as when pro- duced in a fimilar manner by variolous matter. The only difference which I perceived was, in the ftate of the limpid fluid arifing from the action of the virus, which affumed rather a darker hue, and in that of the efflorefcence fpreading round the incifions, which had more of an eryfi- pelatous look than we commonly perceive when variolous matter has been made ufe of in the fame manner; but the whole died away (leaving on the inoculated parts fcabs and fubfequent efchars) without giving me or my patient the leaft trouble.

Figure 4.1. Continued.

[34]

In order to afcertain whether the boy, after feeling fo
flight an affection of the fyftem from the Cow-pox virus,
was fecure from the contagion of the Small-pox, he was
inoculated the ift of July following with variolous matter,
immediately taken from a puftule. Several flight punctures
and incifions were made on both his arms, and the matter
was carefully inferted, but no difeafe followed.   The fame
appearances were obfervable on the arms as we commonly
fee when a patient has had variolous matter applied, after
having either the Cow-pox or the Small-pox. Several months
afterwards, he was again inoculated with variolous matter,
but no fenfible effect was produced on the conftitution.

Here my refearches were interrupted till the fpring of the
year 1798, when from the wetnefs of the early part of the
feafon, many of the farmers' horfes in this neighbourhood
were affected with fore heels, in confequence of which the
Cow-pox broke out among feveral of our dairies, which
afforded me an opportunity of making further obfervations
upon this curious difeafe.

Figure 4.1.   Continued.

[35]

A mare, the property of a perfon who keeps a dairy in a neighbouring parifh, began to have fore heels the latter end of the month of February 1798, which were occafionally wafhed by the fervant men of the farm, Thomas Virgoe, William Wherret, and William Haynes, who in confequence became affeфed with fores in their hands, followed by inflamed lymphatic glands in the arms and axillæ, fhiverings fucceeded by heat, laffitude and general pains in the limbs.   A fingle paroxyfm terminated the difeafe; for within twenty-four hours they were free from general indifpofition, nothing remaining but the fores on their hands.   Haynes and Virgoe, who had gone through the Small-pox from inoculation, defcribed their feelings as very fimilar to thofe which affeфed them on fickening with that malady.   Wherret never had had the Small-pox. Haynes was daily employed as one of the milkers at the farm, and the difeafe began to fhew itfelf among the cows about ten days after he firft affifted in wafhing the mare's heels.   Their nipples became fore in the ufual way, with blueifh puftules; but as remedies were early applied they did not ulcerate to any extent.

Figure 4.1.   Continued.

No. 2

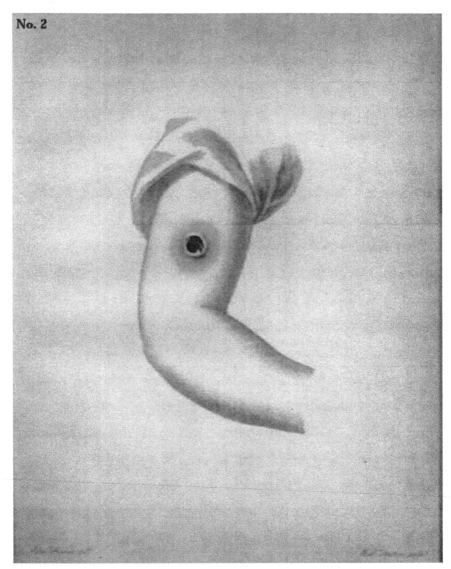

Figure 4.1.   Continued.

[37]

We have feen that the virus from the horfe, when it proves infectious to the human fubject is not to be relied upon as rendering the fyftem fecure from variolous infection, but that the matter produced by it upon the nipple of the cow is perfectly fo. Whether its paffing from the horfe through the human conftitution, as in the prefent inftance, will produce a fimilar effect, remains to be decided. This would now have been effected, but the boy was rendered unfit for inoculation from having felt the effects of a contagious fever in a work-houfe, foon after this experiment was made.

CASE XIX.

WILLIAM SUMMERS, a child of five years and a half old was inoculated the fame day with Baker, with matter taken from the nipples of one of the infected cows, at the farm alluded to in page 35. He became indifpofed on the 6th day, vomited once, and felt the ufual flight fymptoms till the 8th day, when he appeared perfectly well. The progrefs of the puftule, formed by the infection of the virus on the arm. Although it fomewhat refembled a Small-pox puftule, yet its fimilitude was not fo confpicuous as when excited by matter from the nipple of the cow, or when the matter has paffed from thence through the medium of the human fubject.—(See Plate, No. 2.)

Figure 4.1. Continued.

[38]

CASE XX.

FROM William Summers the difeafe was transfered to William Pead a boy of eight years old, who was inoculated March 28th.   On the 6th day he complained of pain in the axilla, and on the 7th was affected with the common fymptoms of a patient fickening with the Small-pox from inoculation, which did not terminate 'till the 3d day after the feizure.   So perfect was the fimilarity to the variolous fever that I was induced to examine the fkin, conceiving there might have been fome eruptions, but none appeared. The efflorefcent blufh around the part punctured in the boy's arm was fo truly characteriftic of that which appears on variolous inoculation, that I have given a reprefentation of it.   The drawing was made when the puftule was begining to die away, and the areola retiring from the centre. (See Plate, No. 3.)

Figure 4.1.   Continued.

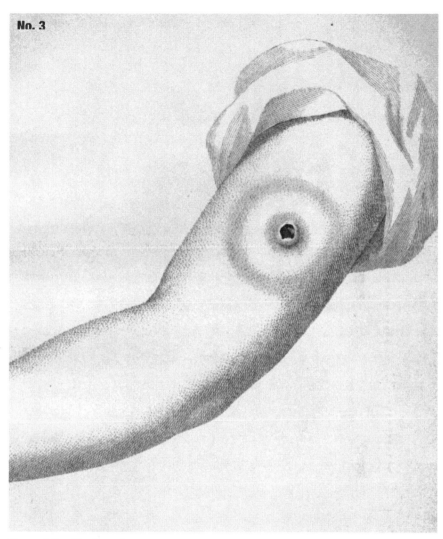

Figure 4.1. Continued.

[39]

CASE XXI.

APRIL 5th. Several children and adults were inoculated from the arm of William Pead. The greater part of them fickened on the 6th day, and were well on the 7th, but in three of the number a fecondary indifpofition arofe in confequence of an extenfive eryfipelatous inflammation which appeared on the inoculated arms. It feemed to arife from the ftate of the puftule, which fpread out, accompanied with fome degree of pain, to about half the diameter of a fix-pence. One of thefe patients was an infant of half a year old. By the application of mercurial ointment to the inflamed parts (a treatment recommended under fimilar circumftances in the inoculated Small-pox) the complaint fubfided without giving much trouble.

HANNAH EXCELL an healthy girl of feven years old, and one of the patients above mentioned, received the

Figure 4.1. Continued.

[40]

infection from the infertion of the virus under the cuticle of the arm in three diftinct points. The puftules which arofe in confequence, fo much refembled, on the 12th day, thofe appearing from the infertion of variolous matter, that an experienced Inoculator would fcarcely have difcovered a fhade of difference at that period. Experience now tells me that almoft the only variation which follows confifts in the puftulous fluids remaining limpid nearly to the time of its total difappearance; and not, as in the direct Small-pox, becoming purulent.—(See Plate, No. 4.)

CASE XXII.

FROM the arm of this girl matter was taken and inferted April 12th into the arms of John Macklove one year and a half old,

Robert F. Jenner, eleven months old,

Mary Pead, 5 years old, and

Mary James, 6 years old.

Figure 4.1. Continued.

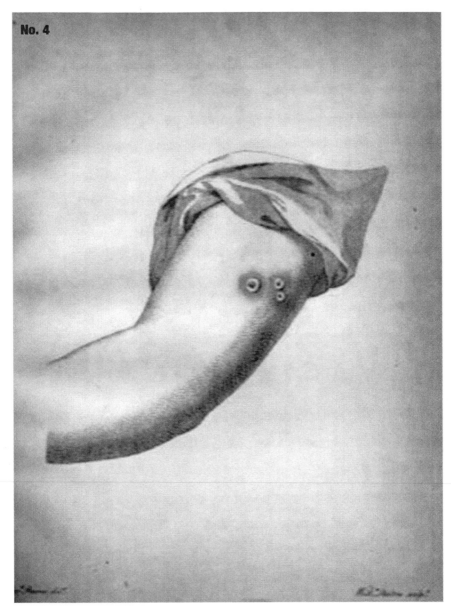

Figure 4.1.   Continued.

[41]

Among thefe Robert F. Jenner did not receive the infection. The arms of the other three inflamed properly and
began to affect the fyftem in the ufual manner; but being
under fome apprehenfions from the preceding Cafes that a
troublefome eryfipelas might arife, I determined on making
an experiment with the view of cutting off its fource.
Accordingly after the patients had felt an indifpofition of
about twelve hours, I applied in two of thefe Cafes out of
the three, on the veficle formed by the virus, a little mild
cauftic, compofed of equal parts of quick-lime and foap,
and fuffered it to remain on the part fix hours *. It feemed
to give the children but little uneafinefs, and effectually
anfwered my intention in preventing the appearance of
eryfipelas. Indeed it feemed to do more, for in half an
hour after its application, the indifpofition of the children
ceafed †. Thefe precautions were perhaps unneceffary as

* Perhaps a few touches with the lapis fcepticus would have proved equally
efficacious.

† What effect would a fimilar treatment produce in inoculation for the Smallpox ?

Figure 4.1. Continued.

[42]

the arm of the third child, Mary Pead, which was fuffered
to take its common courfe, fcabbed quickly, without any
eryfipelas.

CASE XXIII.

FROM this child's arm matter was taken and transferred
to that of J. Barge, a boy of feven years old. He fickened
on the 8th day, went through the difeafe with the ufual
flight fymptoms, and without any inflammation on the arm
beyond the common efflorefcence furrounding the puftule,
an appearance fo often feen in inoculated Small-pox.

After the many fruitlefs attempts to give the Small-pox to
thofe who had had the Cow-pox, it did not appear necef-
fary, nor was it convenient to me, to inoculate the whole of
thofe who had been the fubjeᵴts of thefe late trials; yet I
thought it right to fee the effeᵴts of variolous matter on
fome of them, particularly William Summers, the firft of
thefe patients who had been infeᵴted with matter taken

Figure 4.1. Continued.

[43]

from the cow. He was therefore inoculated with variolous matter from a fresh pustule; but, as in the preceding Cases, the system did not feel the effects of it in the smallest degree. I had an opportunity also of having this boy and William Pead inoculated by my Nephew, Mr. Henry Jenner, whose report to me is as follows: " I have inoculated Pead and Barge, two of the boys whom you lately infected with the Cow-pox. On the 2d day the incisions were inflamed and there was a pale inflammatory stain around them. On the 3d day these appearances were still increasing and their arms itched considerably. On the 4th day, the inflammation was evidently subsiding, and on the 6th it was scarcely perceptible. No symptom of indisposition followed.

To convince myself that the variolous matter made use of was in a perfect state, I at the same time inoculated a patient with some of it who never had gone through the Cow-pox, and it produced the Small-pox in the usual regular manner."

Figure 4.1. Continued.

[44]

Thefe experiments afforded me much fatisfaction, they
proved that the matter in paffing from one human fubject to
another, through five gradations, loft none of its original
properties, J. Barge being the fifth who received the infection fucceffively from William Summers, the boy to whom
it was communicated from the cow.

Figure 4.1.   Continued.

Jenner submitted his findings in a report to the Royal Society of England in
1797. Since Jenner was considered a country doctor, the medical profession
in England rejected his findings and for some time refused to implement the
practice that he had shown to be safe and effective as a vaccination procedure
for smallpox. At this time, scholars did not yet understand concepts attempting
to explain how vaccination could produce an immune protective mechanism
in a patient, thus protecting him from future challenge by the disease organism. More significantly, the cowpox vaccine which Jenner developed could
frequently be contaminated by nurses or doctors who were also working with
patients that had smallpox lesions. Additionally, the vaccination procedure of
Jenner was not always a totally safe one and many children succumbed to the
vaccination, despite the fact that the majority of those treated were protected.
Nevertheless, there was a great outcry from members of the medical profession and also from the clergy, claiming that Jenner's vaccination procedure
was ungodly and un-Christian and should not be permitted. They maintained
that injecting material from an animal was unscientific, criminal, and sinful.

The clergy claimed that Jenner's vaccination method would only work
for those who were not Christians. Since non-Christians in any event were
considered "infidels in the eyes of God" at that time, it didn't matter that they
would be killed by such a vaccination procedure.

Horrifying accounts abusing and criticizing Jenner's vaccination procedure
were circulated, including such vignettes as the following exchange between
an apprehensive mother and her doctor.

Doctor—"Bring your babe now for vaccination!"

Mother—"How you have frightened me, I tremble all over!"

Doctor—"Why? What is the matter?"

Mother—"Pardon me; but I feel a perfect horror creeping over me at the mere thought of vaccination, since my poor Charles has died in consequence of it."

Doctor—"O nonsense! Charles did not die of vaccination; do not believe such a thing. He got dysentery while teething."

Mother—"I beg you to wait another year; Tom is now very delicate indeed."

Doctor—"Only the better! And I have this very moment excellent, fresh vaccine-lymph."

Mother—"In God's name be it done! But, doctor, the responsibility rests on your shoulders!"

Nine days after this conversation and following vaccination, Tom was a corpse, with two vaccine-blisters on each arm.

Cartoons also appeared indicating that inoculation using Jenner's method could result in cows growing out of various parts of people's bodies after they had been vaccinated with the cowpox vaccine, as shown in Figure 4.2.

The procedure for smallpox vaccination developed by Jenner did lend itself to be patented in the early part of the 19th century. Jenner, however, decided not to patent the procedure and essentially made it a gift to the world. The

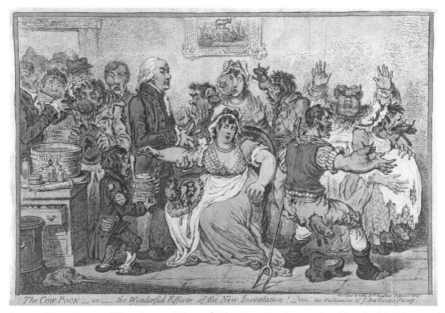

Figure 4.2. James Gillray's rendition of *The Cow-Pock, or, the Wonderful Effects of the New Inoculation!*

term *vaccination* has survived this and related procedures to this day and derives from the Latin *vacca*, which means cow. In a small museum in the town of Berkeley, where Jenner had practiced, the horns of the cow Blossom are on display.

By 1800 most of the medical profession, including most of the countries of the world, had accepted Jenner's work and had implemented vaccination as a routine procedure for children. Jenner received gifts and expressions of gratitude, including statues erected in his honor. Jenner's work won him honors as well as a very generous stipend of 30,000 pounds from the British government to continue his work. The acceptance of Jenner's thesis was strengthened when 70 of the principal physicians and surgeons of London threw their weight behind him. He was elected to membership in all of the learned societies throughout Europe with the exception of the College of Physicians. That group required that he pass an examination in Classics, which Jenner refused. His fame had enhanced his prestige to an extent that his personal request to Napoleon to release a number of British prisoners of war during the war between Britain and France was honored by Napoleon.

The vaccination for smallpox and the courage that Jenner and his associates showed in risking the health and lives of their patients in attempting to find a preventative for the disease in time proved highly successful. In 1980, the International World Health Organization announced that smallpox had literally been obliterated from the face of the earth, and it would no longer be necessary to vaccinate for smallpox. This was a unique achievement; only smallpox vaccination has been able to claim such effectiveness in eradicating an infectious disease.

Jenner died in Berkeley at the age of 74 on January 26, 1823.

Chapter Five

The Renaissance of Italian Research

A superbly detailed compilation by Paula Findlen (1994) has examined the rise of natural philosophy in the 16th and 17th centuries. It shows how the vibrant interest in phenomena of plants, animals, and man were examined and even documented in museums, serving as a precursor to the following centuries when scientific investigation began to blossom. Understanding the socio-economic and religious cultures that prevailed in the 16th and 17th centuries explains to a large degree why Italy, and more particularly the areas where the major Italian universities were built, became a center for scientific investigation.

Up to the time of the early 1800's, a considerable amount of investigation took place primarily in Italy in attempting to understand how certain diseases occur, and how certain diseases can affect healthy people who may have been in contact with a person who was diseased. Contemporaneously, controversy was raging over Jenner's work with smallpox vaccination. Despite the furor, Enrico Acherbe, in 1822, working in Milan, offered the hypothesis that any living parasite, although little understood and not specifically identified, when transmitted from an infected person to a healthy person could reside there, multiply, and then communicate its parasitic character to healthy people. Both the amount of time required for infection to spread from infected people to healthy people and the severity of the disease would depend in part upon the specific disease itself. Since any infectious organisms would be organized bodies that would propagate themselves with those characteristics, they had to grow in the body or in specific organs.

In explaining the geographical epidemics where diseases having similar characteristics would occur, Acherbe theorized that the disease organism had to be something living that could be transmitted from an unhealthy person to a healthy person. Further, it was clear that most people at that time were relatively poor, lived in houses that were rarely cleaned, and wore clothes that were not periodically washed. The nutrition of the general population was such that it would be conducive to the entrance of an infectious parasite that caused disease.

It was therefore not surprising to have been reported that when church dignitaries in England changed the garments of a dead prelate, in order to prepare him for burial, the action uncovered a swarm of fleas and other parasites living in the clothing and on the skin of the prelate. These parasites were quick to leave the dead body and find their way to those standing around the corpse.

Despite the efforts of Acherbe and others, there still remained a large group of scientists and medical people as well as philosophers who felt that spontaneous generation was the mechanism by which organisms availed themselves of the human body and caused disease.

Thus, Acherbe recognized that parasites may be very small, or certainly microscopic in size, and perhaps some even smaller than microscopic. He felt that these lower classes of living organisms belonged to the vegetative (plant) realm of science. Acherbe's conclusions read as if he might have had an insight into organisms so small that they were what we recognize today to be viruses. He wrote:

> These species need the help of particular causes so that their germs will develop and start exercising that vitality which before they only had in theory and not in fact. As these beings start developing, others will form and will detach from the original ones which have given birth to similar beings until all the necessary circumstances stop their development; there their life will stop as well and generation will be suspended within that species and the germs which are leftover will be in a state of latent life that will become active with the reproducing of the same circumstances.

It is remarkable that as early as 1822 Acherbe, in studying petechial fever disease, and without even being able to isolate and identify the organisms involved, was able to elaborate the concept that diseases are caused by living organisms when they propagate to satisfy their own needs to the detriment of the host they invade. Otherwise, no disease can or will occur. Utilizing the concept, Archerbe was able to document the current investigative research of infectious diseases at the time that recognized the presence of commensal and obligate parasites. He was able to show that organisms could survive in a living body without causing active disease if there were no factors to suppress or interfere with their growth.

Acherbe went on to stipulate that disease is caused as a result of contact and that such contact was clearly indicated despite the fact that the identity of disease-causing organisms was unknown and never even identified by him.

Acherbe postulated that these parasites might be microscopic or even sub-microscopic. Their small size, he theorized, in no way detracted from their actions as living pathogens. This was in contrast to concepts of spontaneous generation still held at that time.

The proof of the causal relationship of infectious microorganisms and the pathology they could inflict on healthy bodies was clearly defined over many years of painstaking research by a young lawyer turned scientist, Agostino Bassi.

Chapter Six

Agostino Bassi

"When facts talk, reason is silent because reason is the daughter of fact, but fact is not the son of reason."

—Agostino Bassi

Agostino Bassi,[1] as shown in Figure 6.1, was born a twin on September 25, 1773, from parents who were essentially peasants in the village of Mairago four miles from Lodi in the region of Lombardy. Bassi's mother was Rosa Sommariva. She was the sister of Giovanni Batta Sommariva, a relationship that would serve to improve Bassi's economic standing later in life. His father was Onorato.

During Bassi's youth, his parents had moved to Lodi where they were in charge of a plantation in Mairago. It is not known whether his parents owned the plantation or were merely renting it, but during Agostino's early years, he helped his parents work the land. They grew potatoes and raised sheep.

Once Agostino finished studying in the local gymnasium (high school), his parents had to decide on his further course of education. His father was adamant that his son would study law. Agostino's expressed interest, though, was in the sciences, and ostensibly in the practice of medicine. However, a number of restrictions might have been imposed on Bassi had he entered the profession of medicine, likely prompting his parents to encourage him to study law.

Those desiring to enter a university and procure a degree in the sciences would be required to study "philosophy." A designation of philosophy as a course of study essentially included physics, chemistry, natural history, and related areas of science including medicine. It is a designation of the study of the sciences which has survived to this day in the award of the Ph.D. (Doctor

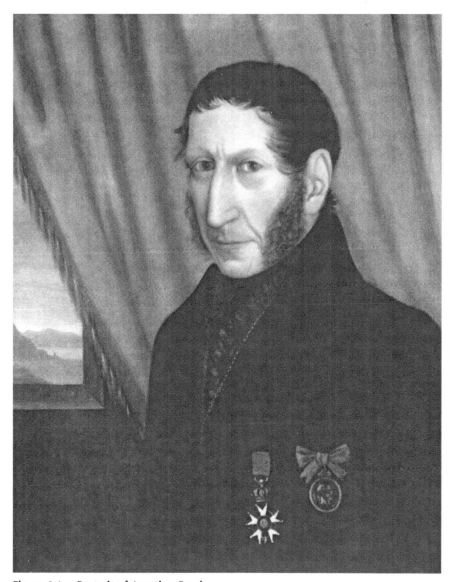

Figure 6.1. Portrait of Agostino Bassi.

of Philosophy) degree, which has for centuries been considered the highest academic degree that a university can bestow on a student.

The system of education at the time Bassi was ready to enter the university was unique to the Italian university system. At that time, the universities conferred only the advanced doctoral degree for the professions of law, medicine, or theology. They did not offer the lower levels of general degrees, such as the Bachelor or Master of Arts degree, (*baccellierato* and/or *magisterium*).

For some period up to and including the early part of the 18th century, the professions of lawyers and physicians had established self-governing institutions called *collegi* (colleges), which had the authority to admit applicants to the university, determine the curricula, and grant doctoral degrees (*doctoratus*). These *collegi* were guilds, as their counterparts were characterized later in a number of other countries in Europe.

The college essentially restricted entrance into the professions of law and medicine to what they characterized as genteel members only. In fact, these *collegi* made entrance requirements more dependent upon the birth and status of the applicants than on their educational background or intellectual capabilities. This resulted in a system of monopolies which could choose whom they wanted to enter these universities. The *collegi* also could use place of birth and other restrictions to determine where the graduates would be allowed to practice. Thus, those who had been born in the countryside could be excluded from practicing in the city.

Those who graduated as physicians with a license to practice were distinguished from other medical participants in several ways. The physicians were educated in general philosophy, and their practice was restricted to the observation of the symptoms and causes of illness. They were not allowed to perform surgical or other bodily interventions. The treatment of wounds and fractures and the excisions of abscesses were left to the "inferior" barber-surgeons as a manual art.

These monopolistic practices of the college of physicians were slowly eroded by the organization of faculty, who would apprentice members for the professions that were closed to those because of irregular birth or status. Many who now entered the medical profession came from villages and towns that hired physicians and paid them a salary in order to provide free health service for their inhabitants. The state supervisor of medical private practice had the authority of pricing and licensing drugs and licensing surgeons and medical practitioners that may have graduated from foreign universities. The activities of state supervisors came into sharp conflict with those of the *collegi,* who were gradually losing their unrivaled authority to admit students to the practice of medicine and dictate the criteria by which they would be licensed to practice.

The hospitals were all essentially run according to the dictates of canon law and were exempt from any government supervision and inspection. They trained their own barber-surgeons and apothecaries through practice in hospital wards and, as such, were in a position to license these professions outside of the jurisdiction of the colleges.

The parents of Bassi had therefore concluded that the study of law would provide their son a better avenue for legal practice. The practice of law would not necessarily be confined to the area where Bassi was born, nor to the restraints of the *collegi*. Bassi went to the University of Pavia where he studied law, primarily to please his parents. However, his studies also included courses of his own liking, such as those in chemistry, mathematics, natural history, and a number of courses in medicine. He had the distinct advantage of studying under a number of outstanding scholars, such as Lazzaro Spallanzani who taught physiology, Antonio Scarpa who lectured on anatomy, Alessandro Volta who gave courses in physics, and Giovanni Rasori who also lectured in physiology. On May 21, 1798, at the age of 25, Bassi received his doctorate in law at the University of Pavia.

Napoleon Bonaparte seized Italy for France in 1796. The French dominated the political as well as the military aspects of Italy. Bassi was named the provincial Administrator of Police in Lodi, where he had moved his family a few years earlier. Later, he was sent to Leone as one of the deputies in the extraordinary consult of the 500. Once there, he was admitted among the electoral community of "Wisemen." He returned to Lodi and occupied the post of central counselor (chancellor) of the Census Delegation.

The desire expressed by Bassi to remain in Lodi with his friends and relatives was not the only reason that prompted him to remain in Lodi. Lodi had become a great political and intellectual center and provided better opportunities for Bassi to fulfill some of his political assignments and also to pursue some of his ancillary interests in the sciences.

The development of Lodi can be traced to the destruction of the Roman "Laus Pompeia." The town of Lodi itself was founded on August 3, 1158, by Frederick I of Swabia. Frederick was also nicknamed Barbarossa (Red Beard). In 1167, Lodi joined the Lombard League. Lodi aided the League in the battle of Legnano in 1176. From 1251 on, many noble families ruled in Lodi, such as the Vistarini, Visconti, and Vignati. Lodi was annexed to Piacenza, but in the 15th century the town was absorbed by Milan and was involved in the battles that Milan fought against the Republic of Venice. In 1413 Pope John and Emperor Sigismund summoned the future Council of Constance from Lodi. At the castle situated in Porta Regale, the local seat of Count Francesco Sforza, the Italian regional States signed the famous Treaty of Lodi, which guaranteed 40 years of political stability. In the years to come, Lodi was absorbed politically and militarily by Spanish, Austrian, and French forces. However, on May 10, 1796, Napoleon defeated the Austrian Marshall Beaulieu, which was the first step of Napoleon's conquest of Milan.

The intellectual and political stability of Lodi thereafter resulted in many people distinguishing themselves, such as Maffeo Vegio who was a humanist, the Piazzas who were a famous dynasty of painters, and the famous playwright and poet Francesco De Lemene.[2]

During this period, Bassi's eyesight had become very weak, and so he had to abandon public jobs and all literary occupations in order to avoid becoming completely blind. To avoid boredom and melancholy, and also to support his family—including himself, his elderly father, a younger brother, and a sister—he decided to take care of the family's agricultural business. Since 1806, he had bought a few dozen expensive Merino sheep. Raising them was advantageous in the beginning, but later on it became uneconomical. A selected flock of 400 or more animals, not counting those he had sold, was the fruit of his great care and unending labor. But this business did not result in any profit, and it actually was so much in debt that he had to abandon it almost completely in 1816.

Political events and a change of government caused the end of the wool trade and also of his precious animals. Bassi, despite great financial loss, insisted on keeping them for a few years. He had hoped that a new government would result in their revaluation, but complete financial need forced him to sell them all to the butchers for a few lire a head. He even had to sell the rams, which he had kept as a treasure for improving the species and for their fine wool. In 1812, Bassi had published an extensive monograph on the raising of sheep.[3] Among the many innovations about which he wrote was his method of turning white the wool of the lambs that were born colored. He also reported a method for getting rid of the horns in the species in a few generations. Bassi also reported on his success at inducing the females to have twins frequently. His monograph on the raising of sheep was published in the *Annals of Agriculture of the Kingdom of Italy.*

Bassi's eyesight improved somewhat during his agricultural work. In 1808, the Minister for Culture offered him the job of administrator of the city hospitals of Lodi at the yearly stipend of 8,000 Italian lira. Before Bassi started that job with the Congregations of Charity, the Minister for Culture asked him to join a committee to direct and administer all the holy places in Lodi. For several years, Bassi had been in charge of such holy places without endangering his eyesight, and therefore he desired to return to his public offices. Consequently, when an administrative delegation was instituted in the city of Lodi in 1815, Bassi volunteered his services. However, after thirteen months of work, his eye disease worsened considerably. It deprived him of his vision for some time, and it never again allowed him to return to perfect health. Thereafter, he was usually restricted from literary occupations.

In 1817, Bassi displayed his enormous versatility by publishing a treatise on the growing of potatoes. In this piece, he described ways that he had developed for planting and picking this useful root on a large acreage. This work was printed by typograph by Giovanni Pallavicini in Lodi under the title *On the Utility and Use of Potatoes and the Best Way of Growing Them.* (Bassi, 1817)

Competition between the winemakers in Italy and those in France began to intensify in the early 1800's. Publications appearing in both countries on methods of winemaking prompted Bassi to publish his own experiences in making wine entitled *A Reminder on the New Methods of Wine Making.* This work was published in Lodi by Giovanni Battista Orcesi in 1823 and later republished in the *Biblioteca Italiana*, Volume 32, page 84. Bassi's reports included not only the preparation of wines from grapes, but also—for the first time in the experience of the winemakers in Europe—the making of wines from various other fruits such as cherries and oranges. Bassi's research included methods of fermentation and aging, and these reports were further published in the *Bioblioteca Italiana*, Volume 35, page 359.

In 1824, Bassi published a monumental analysis of the works of Count Carlo Verri concerning the criteria for growing and fermenting grapes that would lead to a desirable wine. This discourse demonstrates the deep understanding and detailed analysis of the research that Bassi performed over many years. It shows his understanding and use of the best methods of pruning the vines of grapes, the methods of studying the advantages or disadvantages of mixing grapes from different sites to procure a wine having a quality that was desirable, and the best times for planting and spacing of the vines. His decisions depended on many factors, including the specific sites upon which the grapevines were planted.

Bassi taught that grapes, if picked before they are completely ripe, will contain a larger proportion of yeast and less sugar. Consequently, this practice will produce a wine which is improved in that it will be more alcoholic and richer in the concentration of carbonic acid than a wine which could be produced if ripeness had increased prior to picking and fermentation. If the mass of grapes that have been collected to ferment is a large one, then the temperature of the mass would be higher than if the mass were much smaller. A large mass of fermenting grapes leads to a greater composition of sugar and a greater formation of alcohol. However, the increased heat of the enlarged mass of grapes also increases evaporation and the volatility of the alcohol.

Bassi clearly teaches in this monograph that there is an advantage in adding any sugar in small portions during wine fermentation. It was known that sugar is made up of oxygen, carbon, and hydrogen. Bassi explained that the oxygen during fermentation will combine with the carbon of the sugar to form carbonic acid gas and hydrogen. He observed that the fermentation had become impoverished of oxygen and the carbon made for a greater concentration of alcohol, which is desirable during the fermentation. By this observation,

Bassi clearly understood that fermentation that is effected at a lower oxygen availability would therefore increase the amount of alcohol, while fermentation that is provided with a greater degree of oxygen during the fermentation will result in a smaller concentration of alcohol. This knowledge was later acquired and taught by Louis Pasteur and became known as the "Pasteur effect," an observation made by Bassi many years before any work was undertaken by Pasteur to study fermentation principles.

Bassi further elaborated that preserving wine for longer periods of time requires that it be alcoholic. He observed that wines that came from the Lombard area did not have enough alcohol, not because of the species and qualities of the grapes, but as a result of the methods of wine making that provided too much oxygen during the fermentation.

His interest in the fermentation of wine also extended to the methods of manufacturing and aging cheeses. When Count Barni Corrado, a dignitary of the king, established a cheese factory in the Lodi style in the area—at Roncadello in Gerra d'Adda—Bassi wrote a dissertation on cheese-making. It was printed by Antonio Lamperti in Milan in 1820 with the title *Cheese Factory in the Lodi Style in the Roncadello and Gerra d'Adda Location.* Later republished by Giovanni Battista Orcesi in Lodi, this monograph included important criteria for manufacturing cheeses and the ways in which cheeses could be cured and stored after they were produced. The introduction of these methods by Bassi ultimately produced cheeses in the kingdom of Lombardi that were characterized as being far superior to others and became known as Lodigian cheeses.

In 1824, Bassi was offered the position of Professor of Universal History in the Philosophical Institute of Lodi. He was promised pay in Austrian currency, which would have been very desirable at the time. Because his eyesight had been gradually failing for eight years, he was afraid of losing it completely if he accepted; therefore, he refused the appointment.

In the early 1800s, Bassi became increasingly interested in the raising of silkworms.

The silkworm industry is reputed to have originated in China with estimates ranging as far back as 8,000 years ago. The secret of silk manufacture was closely guarded by the Chinese, who exported silk in yarn or in the form of raw silk. The costs were exorbitant and silk generally could only be afforded by the clergy and the nobility. Over the years, India acquired the knowledge of silk manufacture and this knowledge also extended into Persia and finally into Central Asia, including Japan and Korea.

In the sixth century, the Byzantine emperor, Justinian, reportedly came to an arrangement with two Persian monks who had worked as missionaries in China to acquire silkworm eggs and samples of the mulberry seeds in return for a monetary award. The monks returned from China with silkworm eggs reputed to have been of the original strains that began to be introduced into Western Europe.

The countries acquiring the knowledge for the manufacture of silk kept the processes secret in order to monopolize as much of the silk industry as possible. The cities of Tours in France, and Milan in Italy began weaving silk toward the end of the 15th century. Competition between the French and Italian silk industries was fierce. The discovery of a fungus infection that devastated the silkworm industry in both France and Italy resulted in attempts to find a cure for this infection. It was this challenge that led Agostino Bassi to undertake the raising of silkworms in order to study the disease that was decimating the silkworms and produce a method of curtailing the disease.

Bassi's studies in excess of 20 years conclusively proved that the silkworm disease was due to a microscopic parasitic fungus, the growth of which resulted in a white fluffy coat that engulfed the chrysalis of the silkworm. The experiments that he conducted readily demonstrated the source of the infection and a number of ways that could be utilized to separate infected silkworms from healthy ones. The fungus observed by Bassi appeared to be related to the mold *Botrytis paradoxa*.[4]

Bug-killing fungi have been known since 1835, when the entomologist Agostino Bassi realized that the muscardine disease then turning legions of Italy's silk-worms into white mummies was caused by a fungus that could penetrate their shells. The fungus, which grows in soil all over the world, was later named for him.

In the first study being reported today, scientists from Imperial College and the University of Edinburgh sprayed oil containing *Beauveria bassiana* fungus into cardboard pots. Mosquitoes that had taken blood meals were put into the pots for six hours, about the minimum time that they usually rest on a sprayed wall to digest before flying outside to lay eggs.

Many mosquitoes died within 14 days, which is crucial because it takes the malaria parasite about that long to move from the mosquito's abdomen into its saliva so it can be transmitted. Also survivors seemed to fly poorly and bite less, and the parasites in them seemed to develop more slowly, the study said.

That team picked *Beauveria bassiana* because it has already been approved by Western environmental agencies for aphids and whiteflies on melon and tomato crops, Dr. Thomas said, so there is abundant evidence that it is relatively safe for humans, because human bodies are too warm for it to grow in.

Bassi felt that his discoveries of the causative agent of the silkworm disease and the methods of preventing the disease could have significant practical and monetary value. He had fallen on bad times, so he held back publicizing the results of his research, hoping to sell the rights to these discoveries. However, no one came forward to purchase the rights to his research. Therefore, Bassi decided to approach the University of Pavia for permission to communicate some of his experiments and findings, for which purpose a certified commission would dignify the validity of his results. The published announcement of the commission indicated that:

> Signor Doctor Bassi of Lodi in 1833 applied to the Imperial Royal University of Pavia for permission to communicate some of his experiments and findings on the disease of the silkworm called *il segno*. But because during that year the appropriate experiments could not take place, he renewed his application during the current year, 1834. He conducted the experiments in the presence of a Commission composed of members of the faculties of Medicine and Philosophy. Bassi began his lecture by presenting the metamorphosis of the silkworm from the egg to the removal of the silk. The Commission reached the following conclusions:
>
> 1. The white substance, crust, or efflorescence on the silkworm is indeed infectious, and hence placed in contact with a healthy insect will transmit and propagate the disease.
> 2. The efficacy of this substance can be destroyed by various chemical agents which do not damage the insect. This can be done before the said substance is brought into contact with the insect or after, provided the remedy is applied soon after contamination.
> 3. In view of the extreme ease with which this infectious substance spreads, and adheres to everything firmly; and considering the minute size of its particles in consequence of which a single dead worm when reduced to the state of efflorescence can infect a whole silkworm nursery, it cannot be doubted that the said substance is the usual cause of the mentioned disease.
> 4. Seeing that there are chemical agents that can decompose and destroy the infectious substance, the Commission declares its conviction that by the proper use of these agents the all too easy transmission of the disease con be stopped and the disease cured and prevented.

—Dr. Cesare Ripari, Registrar[5]

A signed certificate issued by the archivist of the University of Pavia, 30 August 1834, to verify Bassi's experiments on silkworm disease is shown in Figure 6.2.

The demonstration that had been accepted by the special commission at the University of Pavia resulted in the university issuing a certificate confirming his work. The certificate was printed as the initial preface to both of his volumes published in 1835. The first volume describes the experimental designs he had engaged in, confirming the causative agents of the disease; the second volume describes the methods of preventing the disease from perpetuating itself. Bassi's research set forth the following:

The adult stage of the moth is devoted to the reproductive stage, where the adult males mate with the females that lay eggs. The moths cannot take flight and are unable to consume any nutrition because they have no functional mouth parts.

The eggs laid by the female moth are quite small and resemble in size the seed of a size of a pin head and color of a poppy seed. The eggs will hatch in about two weeks liberating a larva, which is called the silkworm. The silkworm primarily feeds on leaves of the mulberry tree. As it grows, the silkworm undergoes a series of molts. Prior to the 4th molt of the silkworm, the silkworm begins to spin a cocoon by extruding a very fine thread from each of two glands, one on each side of the body. The silkworm will fasten one end of the filaments to a branch or tree and begin to spin the silk thread encircling itself with a continuous thread of approximately 1,000 yards in length. After about 14 days, the larva develops into a pupa stage. The pupa develops a brown hard shell, the chemical structure of which is chitin. The final metamorphosis of the pupa will result in a moth which will emerge from the cocoon. In approximately 14 days, the pupa will emerge from the cocoon as a moth by forcing its way through the silk threaded cocoon surrounding it.

In order to avoid disrupting the continuity of the silk threads in the cocoon, just prior to the emergence of the chrysalis from the cocoon, it is killed by exposing it to steam, after which the thread may be unraveled.

It is relatively simple to recognize the disease *calcino*[6] in silkworms when it has progressed to a state where the infected silkworm is covered with a powdery substance, which can be identified under the microscope as small organisms.

I would take one of the silkworms, still living, that shows the powdery *calcino* covering of this organism, and place it in a clean box. Into this box, I would then place a healthy silkworm that is derived from a box where two silkworms were raised under conditions in which they did not show any signs of the *calcino* infection. They would have been fed fresh mulberry leaves and maintained under conditions which I will describe later to protect against infection from outside sources. The one silkworm that is left behind in the box is removed from the room and continued to be fed until its maturation into a chrysalis or cocoon during which period it shows no sign of any *calcino* infection. The silkworm that was placed into a box with a clearly infected silkworm begins to develop signs of the *calcino* powdery infection in approximately 10 days; after approximately 14 days, it succumbs to the infection being completely covered with the powdery *calcino* dust which consumes the organism, which then dies. The details of the powdery *calcino* can best be seen with an Amici microscope (Bassi, 1837).

In vitro studies of the organism *Botrytis bassiana* utilizing the Amici microscope by Angelo Angelo Cominzoni taken from the reports of Agostino Bassi of Lodi in his report to The Department of Agriculture of Verona dated 31, August 1837 as shown in Figure 6.3.

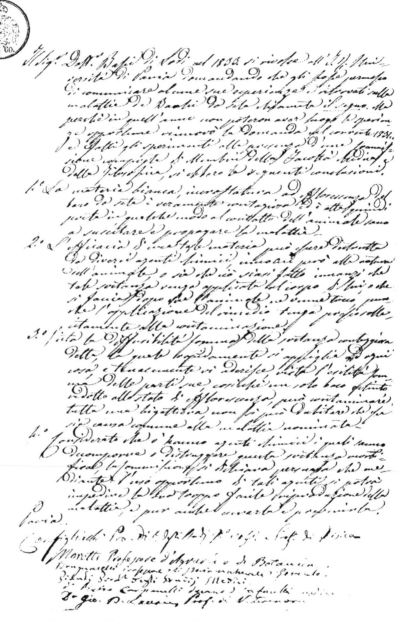

Figure 6.2.   Bassi's research is authenticated by a commission.

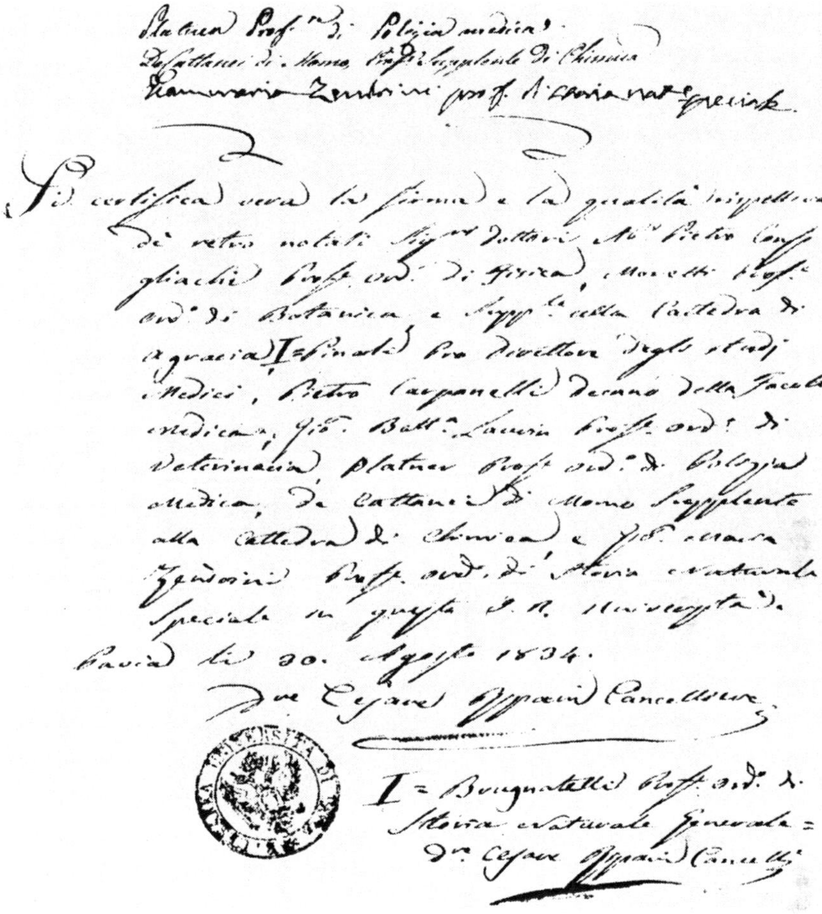
Platner Prof.re di Polizia medica.
De Cattanei di Momo Prof. Supplente di Chimica
Giammaria Zendrini prof. di storia nat. speciale

Si certifica vera la firma e la qualità rispettiva
de' retro notati Sig.ri Dottori: M.r Pietro Confi-
gliachi Prof. ord. di Fisica, Moretti Prof.
ord. di Botanica e Supp.te alla Cattedra di
agraria = Rinaldi Pro Direttore degli studj
Medici, Pietro Campanelli Decano della Facoltà
medica; Gio. Batt.a Lauria Prof. ord. di
Veterinaria, Platner Prof. ord. di Polizia
medica, De Cattanei di Momo Supplente
alla Cattedra di Chimica e Gio. Maria
Zendrini Prof. ord. di Storia Naturale
Speciale in questa I. R. Università.

Pavia li 30. Agosto 1834.

Dr Cesare Oppizzi Cancelliere

I = Brugnatelli Prof. ord. di
Storia naturale Generale =
Dr. Cesare Oppizzi Cancell.re

Figure 6.2. Continued.

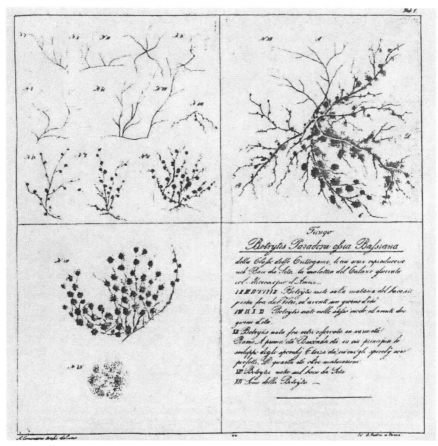

Figure 6.3. Bassi identifies the organism of silkworm disease.

Bassi continues:

It is therefore appropriate and proper to conclude that the healthy silkworm acquires the infection of the *calcino* organism due to contact with an infected silkworm, and that as long as proper conditions to avoid exposure to the *calcino* organism are taken, the silkworms can mature in good health and provide the silk required from the cocoon.

I have performed such an experiment four or five times, and have found in every case that the silkworm that is maintained under good conditions and fed fresh mulberry leaves, free of any contamination, survives in good health and provides good silk from the cocoon. I have also found that the healthy silkworm placed next to an infected silkworm always acquires the disease and dies.

In order to demonstrate that it is not necessary to acquire the infection by close association with a previously infected silkworm, I have removed a dead silkworm which had been clearly infected with the *calcino* organism from the box, destroying it by placing it into a fire, and repeated the experiment by moving a healthy silkworm into the box, whereas a second healthy silkworm was placed into the second box and removed from the room where the *calcino* infection had taken place. After the same period of time, I found that the healthy silkworm, when placed in a box which had previously housed an infected silkworm, acquires a coat of powdery infectious organisms and ultimately is overcome by the organism and will die providing no mature chrysalis from which silk can be procured. Again, the silkworms that have not thus been exposed survive, are healthy, and produce good silk. It is therefore possible to conclude that the presence of the powdery infectious organism that causes the *calcino* disease in silkworms can produce the disease without the necessity of direct contact with an infected silkworm.

In order to understand the way in which the contamination of *calcino* can be transmitted from one silkworm to another, I placed two contaminated silkworms in a box and placed two healthy silkworms in boxes placed on either side of the contaminated box in which all three boxes touched each other. Within five to seven days it was possible to see that the healthy silkworms began to develop a white fluffy coat of *calcino* infection. Ultimately they succumbed to the infection and died. Consequently, close proximity of healthy silkworms need not necessarily be in the same box, and even if they are fed noninfected, healthy mulberry leaves, the closeness of the boxes would ultimately result in some of the infectious *calcino* organisms entering the boxes and infecting the silkworms.

Repeating this experiment, except that the two boxes on either side of the box with contaminated silkworms were separated from the center box by two inches, resulted in essentially the same results. It wasn't until the boxes were separated from the box containing the contaminated silkworm by ten inches[7] or more that we found that contamination from the contaminated silkworm to the healthy silkworm did not occur, except under certain rare conditions.

By these repetitive experiments, Bassi has been able to show conclusively that:

1. An infection of the silkworm, which would render the silkworm incapable of providing the required silk, was due to a powdery growth that could be characterized as a mold or fungus when viewed under the microscope.
2. The disease could be easily transmitted from an infected silkworm to a healthy one by contact. The isolation of the organism from the healthy silkworm which thus becomes infected could be clearly shown to have been transmitted by an infected silkworm. The disease could be easily transmitted from an infected silkworm to a healthy one by contact. The isolation of the organism from the healthy silkworm which thus becomes infected could be clearly shown to have been transmitted by an infected silkworm.
3. A healthy silkworm, when in close proximity to an infected silkworm, can contract the disease, which would prove fatal.
4. If there is sufficient distance between an infected silkworm and a healthy silkworm, the silkworm would not become infected.

5. The presence of an infectious organism in a container, such as a box which had contained an infected organism, could act to infect a healthy silkworm when placed in that same box. Consequently, the presence of the infectious organism outside of the body of an infected silkworm was not necessary to act as the infectious organism in causing the disease.

These criteria by Bassi were essentially the first precise observations proving that (1) infectious microorganisms could cause a disease, (2) such organisms, even when removed from an infected animal, could cause the disease in a healthy animal, and (3) the disease would resemble the disease from which animal it originally had been isolated. In time, these criteria became well established. When reproduced by the experiments of the brilliant microbiologist Robert Koch, they were established for all times as Koch's postulates.

Bassi's research report continues:

In order to avoid the serious damage that muscardine can cause, it is necessary not only to be concerned with the deadly organism to prevent it from getting into your own growth room but you also have to prevent, as much as you can, the introduction of the parasite among your neighbors' silkworms. In order to achieve that, you have to persuade them to adopt your same methods to prevent the spread of the disease and try to make sure that they follow these preventative measures. If by bad fortune, *calcino* would develop in one of your growth rooms, it will be necessary for you to sever any kind of communication with people and instruments between your growth rooms and your neighbors'. It would be necessary to close all the openings in your growth room so that when the wind blows in your direction, it will avoid infected particles from blowing in your direction and contaminating your silkworms. Even flies will have to be kept away from your silkworms, because they can transmit the infection from your neighbors' to your own silkworms. The leaves upon which the silkworm grows will also have to be isolated so that infected leaves from your neighbors' do not enter your own growth rooms. If flies could have touched deadly *calcino* powder in some nearby contaminated facility, they could easily make contact among your own silkworms. Therefore, you should also keep the lights dim in your growth room and also in the rooms where you store the mulberry leaves. There are times when you will have to fumigate these rooms with sulphur.

You should also try to talk your nearby growers, whose silkworms may suffer from the disease of muscardine, into putting in practice all of the things that I have suggested in order to stop the progress of the disease, or at least to diminish it. This will serve to promote the well-being, not only of your own silkworms, but also of your neighbors'. One should try to help each other in the use of expenses, since all of you are fighting a common enemy, which is the prevention as much as is possible of the danger of this disease getting into one's own growing rooms. When this happens, the expenses would be much greater and also the danger of losing the silk crop would become great. Meanwhile, in order to be safer, in case the deadly disease is present in a nearby growth room, or in one's own town, it is better to prevent one's workers from becoming contaminated. Therefore, we should not allow them to pick, to distribute, or in any other way to touch the leaves being given to the silkworms. It is also significant that they should not be permitted to touch the worms themselves, nor to transport them from one growth room to another, nor by any other method of handling until they have washed their hands in one of those liquids of which I will talk about in the following chapter.

The growth room should have a number of open areas so that the room will provide more air and simultaneously protect the room from the noon's sun that may be direct and should not radiate on the silkworms. We should not put too many tables in the same room, but keep them at least ten inches apart. It is desirable to keep the silkworm boxes spread apart from each other and also keep the tables spread apart. The silkworms should be fed often. It is preferred not to use artificial heating after the third molting of the silkworms. The natural heat provided should not be less than 16 degrees C. The room should be aerated day and night, especially after 4 o'clock in the afternoon. The silkworms should be fed with fresh leaves that are recently picked and never less than five times a day.

The bedding upon which the silkworms rest should be removed every 48 hours. If the season is dry and hot, the air around the room will be very dry, and the leaves will be ripe and hard, which requires putting some water in receptacles on the floor during the hottest part of the day, in order to increase the humidity in the growth room. The period during June, because of the heat and humidity, will contribute to the propagation of the disease of calcino. Therefore, during these periods, special care should be taken with regard to the feeding times and to the protection of the silkworms from the heat.

Whether the disease has entered the silkworms or not, once the growth cycle of a silkworm has ended, it is necessary to immediately burn the contents utilized in the growth room, including the wood and paper that is used in retaining the silkworms. Such destruction by burning should be done in an open area and as far away from the growth room as possible. It is desirable to burn the contents utilized as quickly as possible so that fresh wood and paper can be introduced into the growth room. The contents used during the growth cycle of the silkworm should be burned immediately in order to avoid any contamination with new and clean objects or new people that enter the growth room for the next cycle of growth.

All of the grates and other objects that have been used in the growth of the silkworms should be exposed for several days to the rays of the sun. They can be placed on the ground or against a wall, which is turned towards the south side, making sure to turn them around several times a day.

After the cycle of growth of the silkworm is complete, the growth room should be carefully swept, and those things both fixed and moveable should be moved and cleaned. Any removable chrysalis or papers that have not been burned should be put under ground or buried in the middle of a manure field which is fermenting.

The operator should wear a long shirt and should cover his hair under a hat, and wear socks and no shoes. The shirt, the socks, and hat worn by the attendants should be placed in boiling water. The operator should wash his hands and his face with a mixture of alcohol and water. The clothing and related objects worn or used by the servants or any people with any access to the contaminated silkworms should also be put in boiling water. These items, such as sheets, pillow covers, bed covers, and any other fabrics that had been in the room that could have been contaminated in any way, should be placed into boiling water and thoroughly washed. Also, all of the instruments that have been exposed to the infection and also the bags that have been used to carry the leaves and for any other purpose that had to do with the silkworms should be cleaned or burned.

If in the town there are some growth rooms that have been attacked within the year by the disease of calcino, especially if they are nearby, we should avoid communicating with people and with objects from those, not only in the current year, and the following year, but for then all of the time, as long as the disease has not disappeared. For this purpose, we should invite the owner of those facilities, and ask them to take care for their own good and for the good of others, the same precautions to avoid infections of the silkworms. It is also very important to ventilate as soon as possible and as much as one can, all of the rooms, keeping windows and doors open days and nights as long as one can and also make new openings or make the ones that exist already, bigger. Sometimes opening some holes in the corners of the room at least ten inches wide immediately under the roof on one side or the other side of the wall, and better yet above it, helps communicate with the air outside in anyway.

Once the grates have been taken away from the sun, they should be put in a covered place in a well-aerated locale, and they should be put one on top of the other divided with pieces of wood or stones so that the air can still pass to their surface. In March or in April, in which period the germs may be most prevalent and also because the air movement and the intensity of the sun might be diminished, we should purge the rooms, the grates, and the other utensils that may become contaminated. The direct rays of the sun reflected from the bare ground, or by a wall that is facing south, sometimes makes the heat of summer even hotter than 40 degrees or more and sometimes can kill the most hardy germs. The same effect can be produced in several days with lowered temperatures.

Since the grower is never sure to have killed all of the germs that existed on the grate and on the other objects, especially if we consider younger and more resistant germs, in order to be sure of the total extinction of these germs, he will have to resort to other means—the use of boiling water and its steam, a fire of an oven, and especially of the lethal effect of caustic potassium, which by itself could destroy every germ. One can purify the grates with the use of boiling water. A table, which should be longer than the longest grate, should have a rim and a hole cut in it, and the hole should open up over an oven, which is full of hot water. The grate should be placed on top of the table, and people should be at the side of the container holding a metal jar with a strong handle in their hand. They should take the water from inside the boiling oven and pour it several times over the grate until the whole surface of the grate has been wetted. The liquid will flow back by means of gravity into the container that holds the boiling water. This can be repeated over and over again for the number of grates that have to be so sterilized. If one desires to purify the grates by using fire, this can be done with very little expense by hanging beams in an arcade containing four iron wires, and two or more can be attached horizontally at about three arms' lengths from the ground. The grates can be placed over one of the metal wires, and then a number of small canes can be set ablaze underneath the hanging grates. The grates can be turned in order to ensure that all of the sides of the grates have been subjected to the flames. As soon as they have cooled, they may be removed and should be considered free of any contaminating germs.

An excellent manner of disinfecting the grates and other metallic utensils utilized in raising the silkworm can be achieved with the use of caustic potassium. A part of the caustic potassium should be dissolved in eight parts of water, and into this we would add an equal amount of weighted lime that is used in construction.

After a few minutes, once they start losing their strength, they then will be sprinkled several times with this same water, mixing this little by little until the lime becomes a soft paste. A large cauldron is filled with such mix. We then put the grate on the table that was previously mentioned, and one wets it with boiling water. Once we have purged a grate in such a way, we do another one, and then all of the rest.

There is another method, which is not faster, but certainly a little cheaper and all of the growers could use it. It has been practiced by the engineer Pierre of Milan. He puts the lime mix into a large wooden vase, which we usually use to gather and press grapes. Placed into this container, and at an angle would be one of the grates which is made wet with the boiling water all over with a broom so that it will be well-purified. The best method is to form a larger and longer container for the grates, and filled almost completely with the caustic potassium. The grates should be placed within it. As soon as they are wet, they should be taken out and more put in as long as there are some that need to be disinfected. Those that are taking care of transferring the grates into this container also should wear the above-mentioned attire. They should thus purify themselves as we had said when we were talking about the people that have to sweep the rooms. We have to add to this mix a lot of lime and paste, as much as we need to form a thick milky lime substance that is used to cover any utensils as well as the walls of the rooms that have been contaminated, in particular the hot room. This is the room in which the eggs have been placed until they hatch. It is very important to purge this room very well and also the rooms in which the infected grates lay.

We should start by getting the ceiling wet to begin with, then the walls, the doors, the windows, then any of the supports for the grates if they are fixed in the room, and lastly the floor. All of this should be done quickly, and if necessary more people should work at the same time so that after the room is cleaned, it can be closed immediately so that the liquid still is humid on the walls and other utensils in the room, especially the floor. In this way any germs that are in the air and fall to the floor would instead find their tomb as soon as they touch the floor.

While one or more people that are dressed as I have indicated previously are cleaning up the room, others dressed in the same way should treat the glass panes of the windows and wet them if there are any with the potassium that has been diluted, or with the mix of alcohol and water, or with sodium chloride, or with nitric acid that has been diluted. If instead of glass, there was paper to be treated; this paper should have been burned already, as I said previously, with the rest of the paper and wood. With the same liquid, we can disinfect tables, containers, and all of the other instruments that have not been gotten white with the lime. Once all of this has been taken care of, the room should be closed immediately. It should not be opened until 24 hours have passed, or at least 6, making sure that after this, it should be opened as it was before—night and day, as much as possible, especially on windy days.

All of these practices should be enough to purge all of the instruments, but if we want to obtain a total and complete disinfection of the growth room, it is necessary to also fumigate. This should be done once the room is dry after several days with the lime covering which has been applied. Additional purging may be used, especially by those growers that have suffered greatly from the infection the year before and also by those who could not practice exactly the above-mentioned disinfection methods utilizing the caustic potassium. In the rooms that have to be fumigated, we can then put the grates, if they have not undergone the action of the fire, the boiling water, and the vapor long enough; but if they have undergone this treatment, nothing else is actually needed for the full disinfection.

The careful silk grower should study very well my entire considerations in order to keep the deadly infectious seeds away from one's growth room, but also to make it possible for any of the infectious organisms to produce little damage in the case that, by misfortune, they have already entered your growth rooms. Mattresses can be disinfected by rubbing them with a sponge or with a pad that has been wet with raw aqua vitae or with the abovementioned alcohol and water. It is possible to get all of the amounts of potassium that you may require at a moderate price and a very good quality at the drugstore in Milan at Constava ala Palla owned by Mr. Parelli and Paradeezi. If instead of using vases for fumigation, one finds it necessary to spend less, one can use large cobblestones or some other containers as Mr. Cardobeefi of Milan has done, but be careful that they do not crack under the heat. After their use in treating the infected areas, they can also be used for other purposes.

Should one desire to undertake the sterilization of the growth rooms with little expense and with assurance that one would not be making a mistake, it might be useful to be guided at least for the first time by someone who is an expert in both preventing and in curing the disease. Certainly in order to assure one's self that the remedies utilized would not be hurting the silkworms themselves, the owners of this precious animal facility therefore may want to resort, for one time, to the presence of the author of this work. Or if I am not here, someone can be substituted who has been instructed by me in order that they will be able later on to do this themselves and to direct other people to the better advantage of all the growers in general.

If one desires to ensure that they do not make a mistake in preparing the solutions with which to treat the infected areas, and prevent the disease from attacking the silkworms, growers can consult newspapers or some other edition of my work where I have described the exact way to prepare these in terms of the strength of the water and the chemicals that are treated. Growers for now may go to the factory of Domenico d' Egnazio di Belloni in Lodi or to the pharmacist Mr. Siro Stagnoli who lives in the city, and also Guiseppe Basina who lives at 2611 in Milan. They will be able to give you the chloride which I suggest and the nitric acid and the formulas for preparing the appropriate reagents.

Many growers have asked my advice about my methods to treat the infections of the silkworms. I have indicated such information for the benefit of all in the *Git setta priva la jatta* of Milan in Issue 35 of December 16, 1835.[8]

I will willingly come wherever I will be asked to come, as long as I will be reimbursed with one lire for each mile of distance from Lodi and as much for the return trip. As long as the trip, housing, and food will be reimbursed and for that retribution that the owner will decide to give me according to the greater or smaller advantage that this work will bring about or the retribution that will be arranged before. Usually one day staying is enough to receive all of the necessary instruction by me.

NOTES

1. Agostino Bassi in many of his early reports was addressed as Augustin Low, but all of his subsequent research was published under the name Agostino Bassi.

2. An excellent series of reports characterizing those political and philosophical attributes which made the province of Lombardy in Italy a center for research has been written by Elena Brambilla, 1982.

3. "The Well-Intentioned Shepherd" published by De-Stefanis in Milan.

4. This mold was renamed by Balsamo-Crivellis and in honor of Bassi's discovery was named *Botrytis bassiana*. The genus name currently accepted is *Beauveria bassiana*—See McNeil's report in *The New York Times*, June 10, 2005.

5. See Porter (1973).

6. More than one investigator had observed the white filamentous growth on silkworms and therefore a number of terms had been utilized to characterize this problem with silkworms having been called calcinaccio, calcinetto, calcino or muscardine.

7. The literal translation from Bassi's notes speaks of the desirable separation of the boxes containing healthy silkworms from the contaminated silkworms as ten ounces of the Milanese standard of measurement. The nomenclature during the Roman Empire in which standards of weights, measures, and distance were characterized, utilized the

distance one inch, which was equal to 24.58 mm as the "uncia." The uncia means 1/12 in that one uncia is 1/12 of a foot. The foot of 12 inches was described as one "pes" or equal to 295 mm. Since the term uncia has the same root meaning as the weight measurement of an ounce, it is a mistranslation that has resulted in using a unit of measurement for weight the same as a unit of measurement for an inch or uncia. The corrected translation characterizes one uncia as being one inch or 24.58 mm. A detailed discussion of these and related weights and distance measurements has been made by Silvana Iovieno, who was the W & M Officer of Ufficio Provinciale Metrico e del Saggio di Metalli Preziosi of Naples, Italy.

8. A detailed method of Bassi's methodology in preventing infections of the silkworm has been published by Lomeni, 1836.

Chapter Seven

Robert Koch

Robert Koch was born in Germany in 1843. It is generally believed that he was a child prodigy since, at the age of five, by utilizing only the newspapers available to him, he taught himself to read.

He attended the University of Göttingen and studied medicine, graduating with an M.D. degree in 1866. Jacob Henle was professor of anatomy at the time that Koch worked toward his M.D. degree. Koch was no doubt influenced by Henle, who had elaborated and published his views in 1840 that infectious diseases were caused by living organisms.

In 1872, Koch undertook his studies of anthrax, probably as a result of his experiences as a medical officer during the Franco-Prussian War. He set out to determine whether the anthrax bacillus could cause the disease. Without having been in contact with any previously infected animal, he obtained pure cultures of the organisms by growing them in the aqueous humor of an ox's eye. He noticed that under unfavorable conditions, the organisms would become spores and highly resistant to deleterious conditions, such as increased temperature or the lack of oxygen. By growing anthrax organisms for several generations in pure cultures, he was the first to show that they were able to infect animals despite the fact that they had never previously infected any animal.

Koch was able to show that anthrax organisms would normally enter the body through a break in the skin resulting in a lesion. Growth in these lesions could get into the bloodstream of an animal or man, cause a severe bacteremia, and ultimately result in death.

Koch's development of a method to obtain pure cultures of bacteria in 1882 was a great innovation. It made it possible to avoid contaminants contributing to confusion in experiments. Koch isolated bacteria by streaking them on solid media, utilizing a gelatinizing agent extracted from seaweeds called agar. The agar was used to solidify the ingredients for supporting the growth of bacteria. This also permitted him to isolate and identify the organism causing tuberculosis.

Koch also discovered that when the deceased animals were buried, the anthrax organism could go through a metamorphosis and become a spore, surviving for extraordinarily long periods of time. If those spores could be brought to the surface of the earth by earthworms, any healthy animals ingesting the spores would ultimately become ill with anthrax and could die.

These observations by Koch resulted in innovations in the cultivation of microorganisms, first by growing them on solid media such as potatoes, and ultimately on an agar base where the agar had been isolated from certain seaweeds. The technology of being able to isolate bacteria onto artificial bacteriological media is credited to Koch. It opened up the possibility of studying bacteria outside of the person or animal in which they caused the disease. These improvements have been extended over the years and are still used world-wide in order to cultivate microorganisms in the laboratory.

The use of agar as a base for bacteriological media for the growth of microorganisms is essentially attributable to Angelina Hesse, the wife of one of Koch's assistants, Walther Hesse. She observed that agar, which had been used in soups and in other foods, would not degrade at the temperature of 37°C or lower. Agar could be utilized for incubating infectious microorganisms, but could also be melted with various nutriments at 100°C. Such bacteriological media utilizing an agar base, pioneered by Koch and his associates, are in ubiquitous use today for the cultivation of microorganisms.

Koch also pioneered the methods of fixing, staining, and photographing such bacteria. These developments reported by Koch to his colleagues at the University of Breslau in Germany resulted in the publication of Koch's work in 1876. The dissemination of Koch's studies put him in wide prominence among the professional workers studying infectious diseases.

Koch went on to pioneer numerous studies in medical microbiology. These included working with rinderpest disease, characterizing the differences between human and bovine tuberculosis, and studying the disease organisms and diseases caused by trypanosomes and spirochetes.

Ultimately in 1881, he proposed a series of postulates which are still relied upon today to characterize an organism as the etiological agent of an infectious disease:

1. The causative agent must be present in every case of the disease and absent in healthy animals.
2. The causative agent of the disease may be isolated in every case where the disease is suspect and grown in a culture.

3. By inoculating the organisms grown in a culture back into healthy animals, it is possible to reproduce the symptoms of the disease.
4. The agent of disease must then be re-isolated from the infected animal.

Koch became the recipient of world-wide praise and honors. In 1905, he was awarded the Nobel Prize in physiology or medicine.

Thus, when Pasteur began his study of anthrax in 1877, it was doubtlessly the influence of Koch that prompted him to begin his studies on human infections with the anthrax organism. Conclusions made by Koch that the bacillus organism caused anthrax were later confirmed by Pasteur and his co-workers.

Robert Koch died on May 27, 1910, from a heart attack, at the age of 66.

Chapter Eight

Elie Metchnikoff

The Russian scientist Eli Metchnikoff, was born in 1845. Metchnikoff is often considered the "father of immunology." Immunology is that branch of medicine that deals with immunity. The word *immunity* (Latin: *immunis—* free of) was first used in the context of being free of the burden of taxes or military conscription.

In his seminal volume *Immunity in Infectious Diseases,* Metchnikoff reviewed (Chapter 16) the background of those observations by ancient peoples. Through these studies, he confirmed the feasibility of protecting against infectious diseases by utilizing the infectious agent in a small amount or in an attenuated form to produce a state of immunity from subsequent infection.

The idea of a "disease" must have been clear to primitive man. Thus, in the Babylonian writings of Gilgamesh in 2700 B.C., there are records which describe the presence of diseases. Egyptians further characterized a number of diseases they became cognizant of despite the fact that diseases and pestilence were considered punishment by the gods for evil acts of the populations. It ultimately became apparent that once people had been affected with a particular disease, that person, if he were able to survive, would normally be immune to a subsequent exposure to the disease. Thus, the Greek historian Thucydides in 430 B.C. had recorded that the sick and dying received little or no attention. However, those who had already contracted a disease and recovered were recognized for their immunity.

Such observations were made long before the germ theory of disease was postulated. The Chinese are reputed to have practiced immunization circa 1,000 A.D. by making a dry powder from crusts of smallpox lesions and inhaling this powder. The practice was improved in the 15th century by using a sharp needle to insert powdered crusts derived from smallpox into the skin.

This action was taken to avoid smallpox disfigurement, and was primarily practiced on young women whose beauty it was intended to preserve.

De Rochebrune had reported on a type of immunization practiced by the primitive Moors and Pouls of Senegambia (now part of Senegal). The practice consisted of procuring an exudate from the lung of an animal that had died from pleuropneumonia and injecting it under the skin of a healthy animal. The observations that cattle thus treated would not acquire the pleuropneumonia disease have been known since the publication of a pamphlet in Switzerland in 1773 (Rec. de méd.Vét., 1886). Such immunizations of cattle were adopted as a preventative measure in England and Holland towards the end of the 19th century when other attempts to protect against disease failed.

Metchnikoff was a brilliant student, completing the four-year course for a degree in the natural sciences at Kharkov University in just two years. In 1870, at the age of 25, he was appointed Professor of Zoology and Comparative Anatomy at Odessa University.

Metchnikoff attempted suicide following the death of his first wife and again following the death of his second wife, but both attempts were unsuccessful. In 1882, he set up a private laboratory to study comparative embryology, where he discovered the role of certain specialized white blood cells in engulfing any foreign particles or microorganisms, thus destroying them. Metchnikoff called these white blood cells which could digest particles *phagocytes*, from the Greek terms meaning "devouring cells."

In 1888, Elie Metchnikoff joined the staff of the Pasteur Institute in Paris. The discovery of phagocytosis as an immunological method of combating infectious bacteria remained a continuing area of investigation by Metchnikoff. It also prompted a wave of research by many other workers, who began to study similar and related immunological mechanisms that were responsible for removing undesirable particles and microorganisms when they entered the body of an animal. Thus, Kovalevsky studied the phagocytic organisms in the house cricket and demonstrated that these cells would ingest foreign particles that entered the body of the cricket (Kovalevsky, 1894). Aside from these demonstrations of phagocytic activity in invertebrates, many workers began to study the phenomenon in vertebrates. Thus Felix Mesnil (1895) showed that a number of freshwater fish such as perch and goldfish will resist an infection of anthrax organisms. This occurs because leucocytes in the intraperitoneal cavity of the fish attack the anthrax bacteria. They ingest the bacteria and thus inactivate their ability to cause infections.

Robert Koch, in his early studies with anthrax, injected these organisms into frogs. He was able to demonstrate that the frog would have an immunity to anthrax by engulfing these organisms with leucocytes, which destroyed the anthrax bacteria in the same way as had been demonstrated with other animals.

Emil von Behring and F. Nissen (1890) studied the effect of a vaccination on guinea pigs utilizing a vibrios organism (*Vibrio metchnikovi*). Examining the serum of guinea pigs which had been immunized with this vibrio, they found that it was far more bactericidal in inactivating the vibrio organisms than the serum from animals that had not been thus vaccinated. They thus demonstrated that the vaccination of an animal would empower the animal to elicit a protective serum (immune) effect on being exposed to these infectious organisms in the future. Such an inoculation became the mechanism to prevent man and animals from succumbing to infectious diseases. By preparing a "vaccine" utilizing the infectious organism either as is or by its attenuation, the researchers could elicit an immune response to protect the man or animal from subsequent infection.

Another very important observation was that made by the investigator A. Charrin (1889–1890) that it was unnecessary to utilize bacteria either as is or in an attenuated form to elicit an immune response in animals. Charrin observed that although inoculating a rabbit with *Bacillus pyocyaneus* would cause immunity to the bacteria, immunity could also be achieved in an animal by utilizing the products of culturing these bacteria. Such an inoculation into an animal which was devoid of any infectious organisms would still elicit an immune response to the bacteria when the animal was subsequently challenged. This observation was particularly important where the risk of using viable microorganisms in an attempt to produce immunity could provide a great risk to animals and man by resulting in disease. In some cases, it is very difficult to procure an immune response utilizing the organism itself.

One of the early experiments of Metchnikoff would certainly have aroused the interest of Pasteur, who had been charged to study the silkworm fungal pathogen. In 1879, Metchnikoff was the first person to identify a fungal pathogen that might be useful in killing the weevil of grain.

The experiments of Metchnikoff, when he assumed his position in Pasteur's laboratory (see *Virchow's Archiv*, Berlin, 1884), made this very important observation: when anthrax bacilli are injected into a rabbit that had previously been vaccinated, the immediate response of phagocytes in ingesting these bacteria and in preventing a subsequent infection was much more vivid due to the chemotaxic activity of the anthrax bacteria for the phagocytes than when the same amount and culture of these anthrax bacilli are injected into an unvaccinated animal.

Consequently, Metchnikoff showed that vaccination results in a retained immediate response (immune response) to subsequent exposure of the organism, a response which is lacking or very minimal in an animal that has not been immunized.

Although Louis Pasteur rejected this discovery of Metchnikoff, he appointed Metchnikoff as a member of the Pasteur Institute in 1888, and Metchnikoff remained there for the rest of his life.

Metchnikoff observed that many people who drank sour milk lived considerably longer than those that did not. He isolated organisms from sour milk which were identified as *Lactobacilli*. By inoculating milk with *Lactobacilli*, Metchnikoff was able to sour the milk and produce lactic acid. Metchnikoff began to drink sour milk every day to visibly demonstrate how such *lactobacillus* cultures could alter milk to provide lactic acid, and thereby, he concluded, could prolong the life of those who drank it. *Lactobacillus* cultured milk is still sold in quantity on a world-wide basis today. Due to the lactic acid, some of its antibacterial properties in inhibiting certain pathogenic bacteria in the intestinal tract might well be a contributory factor to the concepts initiated by Metchnikoff.

The beginnings of the science of immunology, following the observations and reports of Metchnikoff, certainly had their antecedents in the observations that have already been mentioned. One such observation was that inoculating individuals with small amounts of purulent discharge from lesions of smallpox was efficacious in preventing the onset of a full-blown disease of smallpox. The confidence of observers such as Lady Mary Wortley Montague that vaccinating large numbers of the population would protect them against the scourge of smallpox led her to immunize her own children in this way, albeit a rather crude vaccine by any modern standards.

The observations of Metchnikoff in examining the role that pathogenic organisms can play if utilized as a vaccine—thus eliciting a state of immunity which would protect an individual against subsequent infections—were exactly the conclusions drawn by Jenner in utilizing the cowpox Variola organism to vaccinate against smallpox. Even Jenner had the confidence of his observations to vaccinate his own children, an act which at that time would pose an enormous risk because virology had not yet matured as a science. The discovery of phagocytosis in 1883 by Metchnikoff in demonstrating that certain white blood cells can engulf pathogenic bacteria and thus suppress an infection has also borne fruit more recently in the discovery of chemotactic chemicals such as maltodextrin. When sprinkled on an infected wound, these chemicals will attract the polymorphonuclear leucocytes, engulfing the living or dead pathogenic bacteria and removing them from the infected site. (Silvetti, 1987 and Silvetti, 1993)

Metchnikoff had elaborated the concept of phagocytosis and the role that antigens play in eliciting an immunological response. This made it possible for Pasteur to begin to conduct experiments preparing various vaccines to determine their capability of protecting against infectious diseases.

In 1901, after Metchnikoff completed his monumental book on immunity, he penned a thank you letter to his colleagues at the Pasteur Institute.

TO MESSIEURS E. DUCLAUX AND E. ROUX:
My dear Friends,

Permit me to dedicate to you this work, which sums up the labours of twenty-five years; a very great part of it has been carried out by your side, you who have done so much to lighten my task.

When, nearly fourteen years ago, you allowed me to share your work alongside the venerated Master who founded the House where we have laboured together, you were anything but partisans of my theories; they seemed to you too vitalistic, and not sufficiently physico-chemical. In course of time you became convinced that my ideas were not without foundation, and since then you have given me warm encouragement to pursue my researches in the field that I had marked out for myself.

Working by your side and drawing largely from your vast and varied stores of knowledge, I felt myself safe from those divagations into which a zoologist, who had wandered into the domain of biological chemistry and of medical science, is likely to stray. I thank you with all my heart, and I beg you to accept the homage of this work as a testimony of my deepest gratitude and of my warmest friendship.

ELIE METCHNIKOFF

Institut Pasteur,
3 October, 1901

Simultaneous with the studies of Metchnikoff, Paul Ehrlich was conducting his research in immunology. Ehrlich was born in Germany and obtained his doctorate in medicine in 1878. He became interested in methods of staining microorganisms. His method of staining the tubercle bacillus, an organism discovered by Koch, resulted in modifications which are still in use to this day. In 1882 Ehrlich became a member of the faculty of medicine at the University of Berlin. In 1890 Robert Koch asked Ehrlich to join him as an assistant, at which time he began his studies of immunology. Ehrlich developed the methods of standardizing anti-diphtheria serum which are still utilized to this day. Ehrlich also formulated a theory of immunity in which the side-chains of antigens would result in a specific result of antibodies. Such studies resulted in his being appointed the director of the Royal Institute of Experimental Therapy in Frankfurt in 1899.

Ehrlich's most significant achievement was his study of the effects of various chemicals in killing the spirochete of syphilis. After hundreds of experiments, he found that an arsenic drug, when coupled with a macro-molecule, would be effective in treating syphilis. The compound that he developed, called Salvarsan or compound 606, was in use as the treatment for syphilis until 1940.

In 1908, Paul Ehrlich and Elie Metchnikoff together received the Nobel Prize in Physiology or Medicine for their research on cellular immunity.

Metchnikoff remained head of the Pasteur Institute until he died on July 16, 1916.

Chapter Nine

Louis Pasteur

"Live in the serene peace of libraries and laboratories. . . ."

—Louis Pasteur

Knowledge and its application to achieve novelty, especially in the sciences, frequently can be traced to a metamorphosis of thinking and observations that in relatively small steps lead to major conclusions. Such major conclusions as those enunciated by Louis Pasteur have frequently failed to demonstrate how the precursors of Pasteur laid the groundwork, oftentimes with great clarity. Pasteur would frequently successfully replicate the earlier findings. As has been pointed out by one of his biographers, he would often forget the source of the data for the research he repeated so successfully.

There have been innumerable biographies of the life of Louis Pasteur. Some of the preeminent ones have been authored by Gerald L. Geison and published by the Princeton University Press; Patrice Debré (translated by Elborg Forster) by The Johns Hopkins University Press;[1] René Dubos, 1950 Boston: Little, Brown & Co; and Pasteur Vallery-Radot, 1958 (translated by Alfred Joseph) New York: Knopf. It therefore is unnecessary to detail the early studies of Pasteur and the brilliant studies that he engaged in while studying the racemic structure of crystals. Studying the crystals of a chemical under a microscope, Pasteur discovered that some crystals appeared to be the mirror image of others despite the fact that all the crystals had the same chemical structure. When placed into solution, half the crystals reflected light to the left (levo, or L) while the other half—those that were mirror images—deflected light to the right (dextro, or D).

By September 1852, resulting from his notable experiments and research with racemic acids, Louis Pasteur was promoted to the position of Professor of Chemistry at Strasbourg. He received a prize from the Societi de Pharmaci and a membership in the Legion of Honor.

In 1854, Pasteur was named Professor of Chemistry and Dean of the Faculty of Sciences at Lille. That appointment and the prestige which Pasteur had gained from his research in racemic acid mixtures provided him the opportunity to proclaim that students at the faculty of Lille could do their own laboratory work, for which they would receive a new diploma. This made it possible for Pasteur to utilize these students to assist him in the laboratory studies of his choice.

Pasteur also strongly advocated a strong relationship between the academic faculty at Lille and people in industry to whom he looked for support for his research efforts. Thus when the fermentation of beet root to alcohol was producing products of lower quality than the products previously produced, it was Pasteur who personally went to the beet-root fermentation factory in the area to discover the reasons for the impaired quality of the product. These relationships with industry bore fruit when, in 1857, the directorship of scientific studies at the prestigious Ecole Normale became vacant; Pasteur immediately set out to seek this position. He deprecated the current status of the Ecole Normale, claiming that it required a vigorous new leadership, which obviously he would supply.

Pasteur's skills in organizing laboratories to further his own interests and his administrative skills in procuring funds would lead him frequently to petition Emperor Louis Napoleon for support. He approached the emperor a number of times, pleading for funds so that he could continue his studies pertaining to the contamination of wine and to infectious diseases in general.

Within a few years after his appeals to the emperor of France, Pasteur was able to procure the services of a retinue of research assistants and funds to cover the expenses of his field trips in connection with his studies on fermentation. Some of the income came by diverting funds from the household budget of Ecole Normale. (See *Oeuvres*, VI, pp. 358–369.)

By 1859, Pasteur was able to enlarge his research facilities as a result of his frequent requests for support to Emperor Louis Napoleon. Pasteur's appeals were made through the emperor's aide-de-camp, indicating that the funds would be used for future work on infectious diseases in general. Pasteur also maintained constant appeals to government officials to increase his stipend for laboratory research. In his laboratory at the Ecole Normale, he enlarged his research efforts both for the general study of infectious diseases and for the study of infections of silkworms, which were rampant in France at the time. He now had the services of a bevy of research assistants, and also received an annual laboratory allowance from the French government in the amount of 2,000 francs. Realizing the honors that the French government awarded to Bassi following the translation of Bassi's massive works of twenty years on the infectious nature of the silkworm and how it may be avoided, Pasteur instituted a series of persistent overtures to the French government for additional funds for silkworm research.

The studies of Bassi on silkworm disease and the elaborate experiments that Bassi had performed for approximately 20 years did not go unnoticed in France, where the silkworm disease was beginning to decimate the silkworm industry. Bassi's studies also led to his identifying organisms that caused other infectious diseases. These studies provided Bassi with an understanding of the transmission by microorganisms of human and animal infectious diseases.

The death of Bassi in 1856, as well as Pasteur's overtures to the French government, prompted the French Minister of Agriculture, Jean Baptiste Dumas, to seek Pasteur's help with the silkworm disease. In 1865, he asked Pasteur to undertake a study of the French silkworm blight, which was decimating the manufacture of silk in France.

Thus in 1865, more than thirty years after the conclusion of Bassi's studies on the silkworm disease, after his oral as well as written discourse describing his studies, after his conclusions characterizing the cause of silkworm disease, and after extrapolating from that and other disease organisms the belief that microorganisms were the cause of infectious diseases, Pasteur for the first time undertook to study the silkworm disease. France was producing approximately 26,000,000 kilos of silk annually. Infections of the silkworm chrysalis resulted in losses to the French government of approximately 100,000,000 francs, which at that time, was a devastating amount. Dumas made the request despite the fact that Pasteur had no previous experience with any organisms of infectious origin. Following the request by the French Minister of Agriculture, Pasteur is reputed to have said: "I have never even touched the silkworm."

Armed with the volumes that Bassi had published in 1835 describing his twenty years of research in discovering the etiological agents of the silkworm disease and the methods he had recommended for prevention of transmission of the disease, Pasteur was able to reproduce these experiments. Pasteur's studies of the silkworm epidemic for a period of a few years literally launched his continued studies on the origin of anthrax, rabies, and other infectious entities.

Without formal government support and without an array of assistants being available to him, Bassi had required a total of twenty years to complete his research. Pasteur, provided now with extra funds, assistants, and the French translation of all of Bassi's research efforts, was able to reproduce the experiments of Bassi in approximately five years. In order to immediately publicize the studies that he had achieved concerning the infections of silk-worm and other disease entities, Pasteur founded a new journal. The journal was devoted to the publication of original research papers by his staff and himself in which he proclaimed his understanding and resolution of the etiology of the infection of the silkworm.

Concomitantly with the studies of Bassi on the silkworm disease, Professor Antoine Béchamp, who also performed experiments pertinent to the silkworm infections, had sent a communication to the French Academy entitled "On the Harmlessness of the Vapours of Creosote in the Rearing of Silk-Worms." Béchamp clearly stated: "The disease is parasitical. *Pébrine* attacks the worms at the start from the outside and the germs of the parasite come from the air. The disease, in a word, is not primarily constitutional."

Pasteur had been officially authorized to pursue studies on the silkworm epidemic. In a statement to the Academy of Science on July 23, 1866, he provided a report entitled "New Studies on the Disease of Silkworms" stating that:

> The healthy moth is the moth free from corpuscles; the healthy seed is that derived from moths without corpuscles. I am very much inclined to believe that there is not actual disease of silk-worms. I cannot better make clear my opinion of silk-worm disease than by comparing it to the effects of pulmonary phthisis. My observations of this year have fortified me in the opinion that these little organisms are neither animalcules nor cryptogamic plants. It appears to me that it is chiefly the cellular tissue of all the organs that is transformed into corpuscles or produces them.

The monumental grandiloquence of the positions and statements of Pasteur on the silkworm disease and statements by investigators other than Pasteur prompted Ethel Douglas Hume (1923) to expose the outrageous hypocrisy of Pasteur in claiming to have resolved the etiology of the silkworm. She presented statements and publications made by Pasteur and others to demonstrate this hypocrisy by noting the following:

"Finally, Pasteur went on to contradict Béchamp, in claiming that: 'One would be tempted to believe, especially from the resemblance of the corpuscles to the spores of mucorina, that a parasite had invaded the nurseries. That *would be an error.*'"

Consequently, Pasteur, probably without even conducting any experiments, rejected the idea that there are any parasitic organisms that could be held responsible for the demise of the silkworms. For Pasteur, ultimately, to claim that he had solved the problem of the silkworm disease, Ethel Douglas Hume, by placing the two positions side-by-side and citing the specific references of the comparable statements of Béchamp and Pasteur, has clearly revealed the hypocrisy that Pasteur had demonstrated on innumerable occasions as illustrated by Table 9.1.[2]

Ethel Douglas Hume points out that the early writings of Pasteur on fermentation were consistent with his believing that the ferments could take place *spontaneously*, indicating his essential support for the concept of spontaneous generation. Pasteur, although not explicitly saying so, did tread gently into the arena of accepting some demonstrations of spontaneous generation when he was unable to attribute to any living organism the characteristics of fermentation that he himself observed. Thus, in his seminal paper, "The Physiological Theory of Fermentation": ". . . we are induced to believe

Table 9.1. Béchamp or Pasteur? Who Gave the Correct Diagnosis of the Silk-worm Diseases-*Pébrine* and *Flacherie*?

Béchamp	Pasteur
1865	
Statement before the Agricultural Society of Hérault that *Pébrine* is a parasitical complaint and creosote suggested as a preventive of the parasite.	Statement to the Academy of Science[d] that the corpuscles of *Pébrine* are neither animal nor vegetable. From the point of view of classification should be ranged beside globules of pus, or globules of blood, or better still, granules of starch!
1866	
18 June[a] Statement to the Academy of Science that the disease is parasitical; that *Pébrine* attacks the worms at the start from the outside and that the parasite comes from the air. The disease is not primarily constitutional. Method given for hatching seeds free from *Pébrine*.	23 July[e] Statement to the Academy of Science that one would be tempted to believe that a parasite had invaded the chambers: that would be an error. Inclined to believe that there is no special disease of silkworms, but that it should be compared to the effects of pulmonary phthisis. Little organisms neither animalcules nor cryptogamic plants.
13 August[b] Statement to the Academy of Science describing the parasite as a cell of a vegetable nature.	
27 August[c] Statement to the Academy of Science proving the vibrant corpuscle, Pébrine, to be an (organized) ferment.	

[a]Comptes Rendus 62, p. 1341.
[b]C. R. 63, p. 11.
[c]C. R. 63, P. 391.
[d]Comptes Rendus 61, p. 506.
[e]C. R. 63, pp. 126–142.

that the cells of yeasts, after they have developed from their spores, continue to live and multiply without the intervention of oxygen, and the alcoholic ferments have a mode of life which is probably quite exceptional, since it is not generally met with in other species, vegetable or animal."

Pasteur was ultimately forced to refute the concept of spontaneous generation following the clear experiments of Francisco Redi[3] 200 years earlier, which showed that spontaneous generation was no more than a historical myth.

Pasteur was prompted to examine beer which had become rancid after he was approached by an owner of a brewery in Lille whose beer had turned sour. Pasteur looked at the beer under a microscope and found many microorganisms that certainly had no role in the fermentation of the beer which was attributed to yeasts. Pasteur concluded that the souring of the beer was the result of these microorganisms, but he was in no position to determine how this could be cured. In looking at milk, wines, and vinegar, he also concluded that these liquids were always contaminated by microorganisms and that the microorganisms must be present in the air. By observing that when good milk and wine were exposed to the air, they turned rancid, other researchers reaffirmed Pasteur's conclusions. These were Pasteur's first experiences with microorganisms.[4]

Probably the most authoritative volume concerning the role of microorganisms in fermentation was prepared by Alfred Jörgensen, who was the director of the Laboratory for the Physiology and Technology of Fermentation at Copenhagen, Denmark. (Jörgensen, A., 1900) Jörgensen provided details of the early experiments of Koch in developing methods for the staining and identification of microorganisms. These techniques proved to be extremely helpful in differentiating those organisms which might be responsible for fermentation and those contaminants which might interfere with the fermentation. Jörgensen reported that a considerable amount of experimentation was undertaken by Koch to determine the best methods for reducing the contamination that took place in fermentation, thus permitting yeast cells to survive and carry on the fermentation in producing alcohol.

Jörgensen also reported on similar studies of the use of chemicals and heating to prevent milk from spoiling due to excessive numbers of bacteria. Thus, using a temperature much lower than boiling temperature, including temperatures of 58–62°C, would suffice to kill many vegetative bacteria without destroying the substrate upon which these bacteria would grow. This substrate included milk and other milk products that were used in foods.

Koch also continued to study the effect of various temperatures on reducing the bacterial count of various nutritive liquids, including milk and wines. This process of heating at temperatures below boiling was also confirmed by Koch. These studies by Koch were ultimately repeated by Pasteur, who claimed priority for this relatively low temperature method of reducing the bacterial count of nutritive fluids. Pasteur's persistent claims of priority ultimately resulted in the characterization as "pasteurization" for this technique of relatively low temperature heating of nutritive fluids. It has generally been perceived that pasteurization destroys pathogenic microorganisms as was claimed by Pasteur. It has also been perceived that pasteurization sterilizes milk, freeing it of any microorganisms. This is a myth that has been perpetuated for many years and is totally contrary to fact.

The United States Centers for Disease Control and Prevention, part of the Department of Health and Human Services, promotes the drinking solely of pasteurized milk, ostensibly to deter people from drinking raw milk. In the documents (Morbidity and Mortality Weekly Report—Centers for Disease Control and Prevention—2007), we find the statements that: "Pasteurization is a simple process. In the United States, raw milk is collected from cows and heated to a high temperature for a short period of time. This destroys any harmful germs that may be contaminating the milk."

It is categorically untrue that pasteurization of milk as it is practiced in the United States today, and presumably elsewhere, *destroys* (emphasis added) all harmful germs that are contaminating the milk. Pasteurization may reduce the numbers of harmful germs in raw milk; but the evidence is quite clear that such reduction of pathogenic organisms in raw milk does not destroy their ability to frequently cause disease processes in people who drink pasteurized milk.

Access to the Internet under the title of "pasteurization" also provides the information that: "In pasteurization of milk, pathogenic bacteria are destroyed by heating at 62 degrees C for 30 minutes, or by 'flash' heating to 62 degrees C for less than 10 to 30 seconds. In Norway, the milk is usually heated to 72 degrees C for 15 seconds. The pasteurization process reduces the bacterial count of the milk by 97% to 99%."

Though there is reason to challenge the blatant characterization that pasteurization reduces the bacterial count by 97–99 percent, that statement in this same document is totally inconsistent with the one above it that states that pasteurization destroys all pathogenic bacteria. In a highly controversial book (*The Medical Mafia*, 1994), Dr. Ghislaine Lanctôt pointed out that pasteurization does not utilize a temperature high enough to destroy all pathogenic microorganisms and uses a temperature that is too high to leave milk and other nutritive fluids unharmed. It would appear, therefore, that the documentation that has accumulated over the years sustains the argument that pasteurization does not kill pathogenic bacteria, certainly not in milk. There have been a considerable number of epidemics throughout the years which have specifically pointed to pasteurized milk as having been responsible for thousands of people becoming ill with infections of *Yersinia enterocolitica*, *Salmonella*, *Listeria*, and *E. coli*.

It has not been understood by the general public that pasteurization, which had been developed by Tyndall and Koch and repeated by Pasteur, does not sterilize milk, because the temperature is too low to achieve sterilization. It does reduce the bacterial count so that the milk can be labeled with a particular expiration date prior to which it is presumed that it can be safely consumed, especially if kept refrigerated.

The numbers of bacteria that can properly be permitted in pasteurized milk, at least in the United States, are mandated by the United States Food and Drug Administration. The procedures for performing such counts are contained in publications of the American Public Health Association, Inc., such as that published in the year 1967. There is some latitude for additional criteria of the merits of the bacterial counts for milk from state to state. Basically, however, the following examples of enforcement procedures of the United States Food and Drug Administration indicate the bacterial counts that are permitted in milk soon after pasteurization. The assumption that those counts can be sustained between the time the milk is pasteurized and the milk reaches the dinner table of the consumer has not yet been proved. It will be noted, however, that the United States Food and Drug Administration does permit a quantity of coliform bacteria—which indicates fecal contamination—to be present in pasteurized milk. It would almost bring milk production to a halt if the coliform count were mandated to be zero.

Tables 9.2 and 9.3 provide several examples of the application of the enforcement system described in Section 6 of the United States Food and Drug Administration. While the illustrations pertain only to pasteurized milk bacterial counts and somatic cell counts of raw milk, the method is applied, in like fashion, to the enforcement of established standards for cooling temperature, coliform limits, etc. Pasteurized milk or milk product that shows a positive phosphatase reaction and milk or milk product in which the presence of drug residue, pesticides, or other adulterants are found, shall be dealt with as indicated in Sections 2 and 6, respectively of the code of the United States Food and Drug Administration.

An example of the permitted coliform counts, as legislated in the state of Minnesota, the statutes provide that "Grade A pasteurized milk, fluid milk products, and goat milk are Grade A raw milk, fluid milk products and goat milk for pasteurization which have been pasteurized, cooled and prepared for distribution in a dairy plant approved by the commissioner, the bacterial count of which at no time after pasteurization and until delivery exceeds 20,000 bacteria per milliliter. The coliform count must not exceed ten per milliliter except that bulk tank transport shipments must not exceed 100 per milliliter."[5]

Table 9.2.   Example of Enforcement Procedures for Pasteurized Milk Laboratory Examinations

Date	Bacterial Count Per mL	Enforcement Action as Applied to a Standard of 20,000/mL
1/05/05	6,000	No Action Required
1/28/05	11,000	No Action Required
2/11/05	12,000	No Action Required
3/15/05	22,000	Violative; No Action Required
3/25/05	23,000	Violative; Written notice to plant, 2 of last 4 counts exceed the standard. (This notice shall be in effect as long as 2 of the last 4 consecutive samples exceed the standard). Additional sample required within 21 days from the date of the notice, but not before the lapse of three (3) days.
4/02/05	9,000	No Action Required
4/19/05	51,000	Violative (3 of last 5 counts exceed the standard); Required Regulatory Actions: 1. Suspend plant permit; or 2. Forego permit suspension, provided the milk or milk product(s) in violation are not sold as Grade "A" product(s); or 3. Impose monetary penalty in lieu of permit suspension, provided the milk or milk product(s) in violation are not sold as Grade "A" milk or milk product(s).
4/23/05		Issue temporary permit (if applicable) after plant inspection. Begin accelerated sampling schedule.
4/25/05	11,000	No Action Required
4/29/05	3,000	No Action Requited
5/4/05	22,000	Violative; No Action Required NOTE: Samples collected prior to 4/23/05 are not used for subsequent bacterial count enforcement purposes.
5/9/05	5,000	Permit Fully Reinstated

Pasteur proclaimed time and time again that heating milk to the temperature and for the time period he recommended would destroy any pathogenic bacteria in the milk. This erroneous assertion has been perpetuated in literature and for the benefit of the public in categorically stating that pasteurization destroys pathogenic bacteria. Evidence contradicting this assertion is legion. The mere examination of the records for the Los Angeles County Board of Supervisors report gathered by Dr. Lanctôt clearly documents the plethora of infections and outbreaks resulting from pasteurized milk and milk products:

1997, 28 persons ill from *Salmonella* in California, all from pasteurized milk.
1996, 46 persons ill from *Campylobacter* and *Salmonella* in California.
1994, 105 persons ill from *E. coli* and *Listeria* in California.
March of 1985, 19,660 confirmed cases of *Salmonella typhimurium* illness from consuming properly pasteurized milk. Over 200,000 people ill from *Salmonella typhimurium* in pasteurized milk.

Table 9.3.   Enforcement Actions for Bacteria Counts Allowed in Milk

Date	Confirmed Somatic Cell Counts per mL	Enforcement Action as Applied to a Standard of 750,000 per mL
7/10/05	500,000	No Action Required
8/15/05	600,000	No Action Required
10/1/05	800,000	Violative; No Action Required
11/7/05	900,000	Violative; Written notice to producer, 2 of last 4 counts exceed the standard. (This notice shall be in effect as long as 2 of the last 4 consecutive samples exceed the standard). Additional sample required within 21 days from the date of the notice, but not before the lapse of three (3) days.
11/14/05	1,200,000	Violative (3 of last 5 counts exceed the standard); Required Regulatory Actions: 1. Suspend producer permit; or 2. Forego permit suspension, provided the milk in violation is not sold or offered for sale as Grade "A"; or 3. Impose monetary penalty in lieu of permit suspension, provided the milk in violation is not sold or offered for sale as Grade "A" product. Except that a milk producer may be assessed a monetary penalty in lieu of permit suspension for violative counts provided: If the monetary penalty is due to a violation of the somatic cell count standard, the Regulatory Agency shall verify that the milk supply is within acceptable limits as prescribed in Section 7 of this *Ordinance*. Samples shall then be taken at the rate of not more than two (2) per week on separate days within a three (3) week period in order to determine compliance with the appropriate standard as determined in accordance with Section 6 of this *Ordinance*.
11/18/05	700,000	Issue temporary permit (if applicable) after sampling indicates the milk is within the standards prescribed in Section 7. Begin accelerated sampling schedule.
11/20/05	800,000	Violative; No Action Required Note: Samples collected prior to 11/18/05 are not used for subsequent somatic cell count enforcement purposes.
11/24/05	700,000	No Action Required
11/29/05	550,000	Permit Fully Reinstated

1985, 142 cases and 47 deaths traced to pasteurized Mexican-style cheese contaminated with *Listeria monocytogenes*. *Listeria monocytogenes* survives pasteurization.

1985, 1,500 persons ill from *Salmonella* infection.

August of 1984, approximately 200 persons became ill with a *Salmonella typhimurium* from consuming pasteurized milk.

November of 1984, another outbreak of *Salmonella typhimurium* illness from consuming pasteurized milk.

1983, 28 persons ill from *Salmonella* infection.

IN OTHER STATES:

1983, over 49 persons with *Listeria* illness have been associated with the consumption of pasteurized milk in Massachusetts.

1982, 172 persons ill (100 hospitalized) in three Southern states from pasteurized milk.

1982, over 17,000 persons became ill with *Yersinia enterocolitica* from pasteurized milk bottled in Memphis, Tennessee.

Many potentially harmful effects of pasteurization have been reported by a number of individuals and also by The Weston A. Price Foundation. Publications by The Weston A. Price Foundation have also cited Dr. Kurt A. Oster indicating that homogenization of milk reduces the size of the fat particle, thus permitting the fat particles to be assimilated into the stomach lining. When these fat particles ultimately get into the bloodstream, a defense mechanism is created, resulting in the scarring of arteries.

The author also analyzed the incidence of antibodies in the blood serum of patients chosen at random who consumed milk and related dairy products in relatively large quantities. In a random selective population of 50 specimens so tested, 5 percent showed antibodies to bovine albumen and bovine gammaglobulin. It is not unreasonable to believe that ingestion of milk and milk products can excite the Peyer's patches in the intestine, resulting in hypersensitivity and in some cases anaphylaxis, and possibly explaining the inability of some infants to drink and digest cow's milk.

Jörgensen's monumental study also points out that vessels employed in sterilizing liquids were provided with a series of bent tubes so that their contents would remain sterile. Such vessels were initially developed by Milne-Edwards Chevreul and Hoffmann. They were ultimately prepared in the same manner by Pasteur. An improvement of these initial flasks with bent tubes was developed by Charles Chamberland, who worked with Louis Pasteur. Chamberland boiled the solution in a flask and the vapors would pass out of the flask through a cotton plug. The plug acted as an impediment to any bacteria or particles making their way back into the flask after the medium had been sterilized by boiling for a suitable period of time. This concept of using a cotton plug in a test tube after bacteria had been inoculated therein, with such a tube containing a nutrient medium, has been in use essentially unchanged to the present time.

The flask developed by Hansen also contained a cap with a cotton wool filter and a small-sized side tube with an asbestos stopper. The various swan-necked flasks and their proponents are shown in Figures 9.1 and 9.2. The flask developed by Eduard von Freudenreich is essentially the same as the Chamberland flask except that it was prepared in a cylindrical shape.

Jörgensen (1900), p.p. 19–22 described the various uses of the swan-necked flasks. For the Carlsberg flask, as illustrated in Figure 9.2, the hopped wort

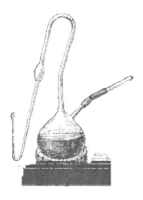

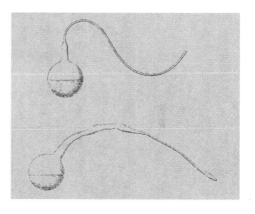

The Chevreul and Hoffmann flask developed at the Carlsberg Physiological Laboratories (Jörgensen, 1900, p.19)

The swan-necked flasks used by Pasteur (Geison 1995, p. 117)

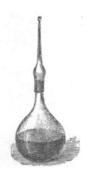

Chamberland Flask

Figure 9.1.   Swan-necked flasks used to repudiate spontaneous generation.

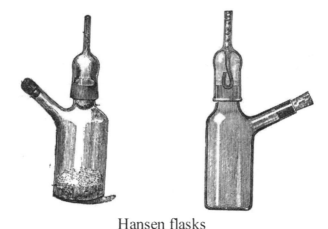

Hansen flasks

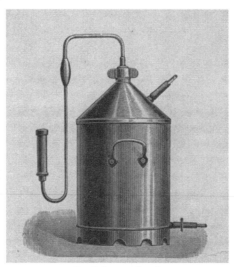

Carlsberg flask

Figure 9.2.   Hansen and Carlsberg flasks.

(preferably filter-bag wort) is boiled, the steam first escapes through the wide straight tube, at the end of which is a piece of India-rubber tubing; when this is closed after boiling (for about a quarter of an hour) the only outlet for the steam is through the bent tube. About ten minutes after, the flask is taken from the sand-bath, and the bent tube may be closed with a plug of asbestos. The contents of the flask can remain for years without undergoing any change.

The Carlsberg experiments with the swan-necked tubes showed that microorganisms could not begin to grow in the sterilized wort "spontaneously" if organisms were prevented from entering the sterilized wort medium due to the configuration of swan-necked flasks.

Geison in his biography of Pasteur[6] indicates that Pasteur was aware that Chevreul had already performed experiments with the swan-necked flasks in his chemistry lectures. (See Duclaux, 1896.)

Pasteur, in his 1864 lecture to the Sorbonne, ignored any precedent with swan-necked flasks claiming that: "Never will the doctrine of spontaneous generation recover from the mortal blow struck by this simple experiment" (referring to his swan-necked flasks experiments, where he showed that microorganisms would not grow in the swan-necked flask containing a sterile fermentable juice).[7] The swan-necked flask of Pasteur can be seen in Figure 9.3 of Pasteur's page 108 of his research notebook. The translation in French of Figure 9.3 is contained in Figure 9.4.

Pasteur correctly concluded that the fermentation of wine and beer was caused by the yeasts in the fermentation liquor and that the bacteria present would result in spoilage to the fermentation. Consequently, he confirmed that heating grape juice to approximately 55 degrees Centigrade would kill many of the bacteria that spoiled the wine without affecting the fermentation to produce alcohol. This heating mechanism was later extrapolated by Pasteur to beer and milk and acquired the name *pasteurization*.

Pasteur's work with fermentations was the steppingstone for him to investigate and study the nature of infections and methods of their prevention.

In 1865 when Pasteur was asked to investigate diseases of the silkworm by the French government, he instituted plans to study microorganisms that could cause disease not only in animals, but also in humans. Thus, in 1865 when a cholera epidemic was raging in Marseilles, Pasteur tried to find the germ that caused the cholera, but was not successful. Since his education and experience had predominantly been in the field of chemistry, Pasteur felt that he lacked sufficient medical knowledge to direct his efforts to diseases of animals and humans. Therefore he hired two bright young doctors to join his team—Emile Roux and Charles Chamberland.

Pasteur was likely influenced by Koch's brilliant development of the methods for growing and identifying bacteria, by Koch's experiments which confirmed the germ theory of disease, and by his experimental findings concerning the disease of anthrax. All these developments might have been an impetus that prompted Pasteur to tackle the infections of animals with anthrax, especially since this disease was very common among the animals raised in France.

Pasteur found that anthrax bacillus injected into chickens did not cause the disease, probably because the body temperature of chickens—between

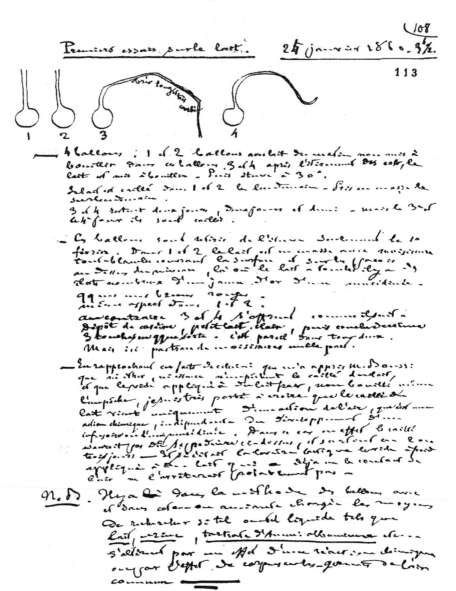

Figure 9.3.   A page from Pasteur's notebook describing the swan-necked flasks.

Premiers essais sur le lait.   2$/4 janvier 1860 - 3 ʰ 1/2.

Très long *et très*
courbé

1   2   3   4

– 4 ballons. 1 et 2 ballons avec lait du matin non mis à
bouillir dans ces ballons. 3 et 4 après l'étirement des cols, le
lait est mis à bouillir – Puis étuve à 30°.
Le lait est caillé dans 1 et 2 le lendemain – Pris en masse le
surlendemain.
3 et 4 restent deux jours, deux jours et demi – Mais le 3ᵉ et
le 4ᵉ jour ils sont caillés.

– Ces ballons sont retirés de l'étuve seulement le 10
février. Dans 1 et 2 le lait est en masse avec moisissure
toute blanche couvrant la surface et sur les parois
au dessus du niveau, là où le lait a touché il y a des
îlots nombreux d'un jaune d'or d'une mucédinée –
qques uns bruns rouges –
même aspect dans 1 et 2.
au contraire 3 et 4 s'offrent comme il suit –
Dépôt de caséïne, petit lait clair, puis couche de crème
3 couches en qque sorte – C'est pareil dans tous deux.
Mais ici pas trace de moisissures nulle part.

– En rapprochant ces faits de celui-ci que m'a appris M. Bouss :
que ni éther, ni essence n'empêchent le caillé du lait,
et que le vide appliqué à du lait frais, non bouilli même
l'empêche, je suis très porté à croire que le caillé du
lait vient uniquement d'une action de l'air, que c'est une
action chimique, indépendante du développement d'un
infusoire ou d'une mucédinée. Dans ce cas en effet le caillé
n'aurait pas dû se produire ci-dessus, et surtout en 2 ou
trois jours – Et si c'était la levûre lactique le vide à froid
appliqué à du lait qui a déjà eu le contact de
l'air ne l'arrêterait probablement pas –

N. B.   Il y a là dans la méthode des ballons avec
et sans coton ou amiante chargée les moyens
de rechercher si tel ou tel liquide tels que
lait, urine, tartrate d'Amm : albumineux etc...
s'altèrent par un effet d'une réaction chimique
ou par l'effet de corpuscules-germes de l'air
commun ⸻

Figure 9.4. Translation of Pasteur's notebook shown in Figure 9.3.

39 and 42 degrees Centigrade—was higher than that of humans. However, anthrax could be introduced into these chickens if their body temperature was lowered by submerging the chickens in cold water prior to inoculation with anthrax organisms.

Pasteur proclaimed that the spores of anthrax would not form at 42–43 degrees C and that the bacteria would continue to multiply. He went on to claim that exposing anthrax organisms to oxygen would yield attenuated microorganisms that would protect such animals as rabbits, guinea pigs, and sheep against a subsequent injection of the anthrax spores.

These particular experiments performed by Pasteur with anthrax were not available to microbiologists, because Pasteur in his will had ordered that his research notebooks should never be laid open to the public. However, one of his heirs donated the Pasteur research notebooks to the national library in Paris. In 1995 Professor Gerald Geison at Princeton University, after a study of Pasteur's laboratory notebooks, reported the following:

> A claim that Pasteur made that exposing anthrax bacteria to oxygen would produce an attenuated vaccine that would protect animals against subsequent exposure was, in fact, a deliberate lie, since the truth was that his vaccine had relied on a technique used by a veterinary surgeon, Jean Joseph Henri Toussaint, which utilized potassium chromate to attenuate the organisms.

Following the demonstration that the potassium chromate inactivated anthrax organisms were successful in protecting animals against subsequent exposure to anthrax, Pasteur agreed to a public demonstration of the potency of this vaccine on June 2, 1881. It did, in fact, demonstrate that the vaccine would protect against subsequent challenge with a virulent culture of anthrax. Pasteur permitted the manufacture of the anthrax vaccine only at his laboratory, thus assuring that he would be in a position to control its manufacture and sale.

Pasteur's laboratory could not meet the huge demand for the vaccine. In addition, many animals vaccinated with the vaccine died. Complaints became rampant, not only in France but also in other countries, that Pasteur's vaccine would not protect against subsequent exposure to anthrax organisms.

The fact that the anthrax vaccine of Pasteur had been contaminated with other organisms was elegantly tested and publicly exposed by Robert Koch. Koch, at a public scientific meeting, accused Pasteur of being negligent in preparing the vaccine. He declared: "Such goings-on are perhaps suitable for the advertising of a business house, but science should reject them vigorously."

Ordinarily such a revelation of malfeasance by a scientist would have ended his career. But the French government was not about to impair the reputation of Pasteur, especially since such a criticism had come from a

"German." It was therefore not unexpected that the French government following these revelations by Koch elected Pasteur a member of the Académie Française, and even the famous philosopher Ernest Renan praised Pasteur as being a genius.

There have been numerous publications attributing to Pasteur the remark that he chose not to patent any of his processes because, according to his credo, "Knowledge belongs to humanity." (See also P. J. Federico, 1937.) As proof that he did file patents, a drawing from the patent by Louis Pasteur for the brewing of beer is shown in Figure 9.5.

Some historians believe that beer was first made by the Sumerians as early as the 4000's B.C. The technology was later absorbed into the Babylonian and ancient Egyptian cultures. The Sumerians baked grains into bread, and the bread was moistened to begin the process of making beer. The baked bread was a way to preserve the grain for later use in the beer making process. A Sumerian beer was recreated recently by the staff at Anchor Steam Beer as an experiment. In more recent times, Louis Pasteur studied beer and wine making and patented a process, for making beer which resulted in a better beer as seen in Figure 9.5. Previously the wort was boiled and exposed to the air for cooling. In Pasteur's process, the wort was kept in closed vessels and cooled by spraying the outside of the vessel with water. A special yeast was introduced into the mash after it cooled, thus preventing contamination of the wort with stray wild yeasts floating through the air.

Maurice Cassier (2005), in discussing the appropriation and commercialization of the Pasteur anthrax vaccine, proclaimed:

> Whereas Pasteur patented the biotechnological processes that he invented between 1857 and 1873 in the agro-food domain, he did not file any patents on the artificial vaccine preparation processes that he subsequently developed. This absence of patents can probably be explained by the 1844 patent law in France that established the non-patentable status of pharmaceutical preparations and remedies, including those for use in veterinary medicine. Despite the absence of patents, the commercial exploitation of the anthrax vaccine in the 1880's and 1890's led to a technical and commercial monopoly by Pasteur's laboratory as well as the founding of a commercial company to diffuse the vaccine abroad. Pasteur repeatedly refused to transfer his know-how and anthrax vaccine production methods to foreign laboratories, on the grounds that he wished to control the quality of the vaccines produced. Indeed, it was relatively difficult to transfer a method that was not yet perfectly stabilized in the early 1880s. Pasteur also wanted to maintain the monopoly of his commercial company and to increase the profits from vaccine sales so that the Institut Pasteur could be financially independent. The Pasteur anthrax vaccine operating licenses are described and analyzed in detail in this article.

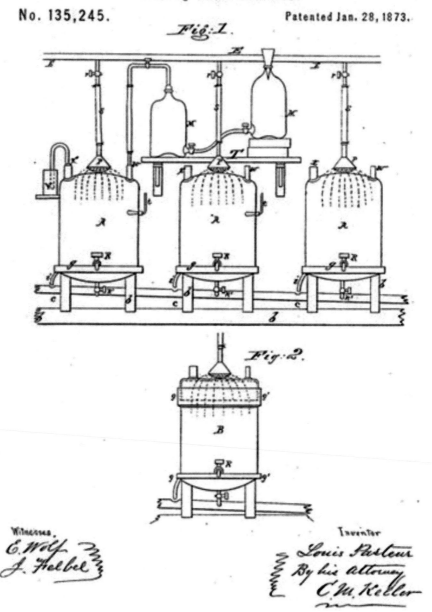

Figure 9.5. The drawing from Pasteur's patent describing the manufacture of beer.

Attenuation techniques that ultimately prepared successful vaccines for cholera and anthrax could not be applied to a number of other diseases, such as the diphtheria organism. It fell to investigators such as Friedrich Löffler, who was a student of Robert Koch, to prepare the toxin of diphtheria by filtering the organisms through a Chamberland porcelain filter that excluded the bacteria themselves. It was thus possible, by injecting the bacteria-free filtrate to show that the clinical symptoms of diphtheria could be reproduced in experimental animals. A relative estimate of the toxicity of the diphtheria toxin was ultimately achieved by Emile Roux of the Pasteur Institute by computing that one ounce of the pure toxin was sufficient to kill 600,000 guinea pigs.

An article by Kendall A. Smith (2005) reported on the studies by Pasteur in attempting to prepare vaccines in dealing with infectious diseases. Dr. Smith's report begins to unravel the mythology which has surrounded Louis Pasteur, in part due to Pasteur's own efforts, and in part due to the role played by the French government. Smith points out that: "In France one can be an anarchist, a communist or a nihilist, but not an anti-Pasteurian. A simple question of science has been made into a question of patriotism." He also quotes Stephen Paget as claiming that "[Pasteur] was the most perfect man who has ever entered the kingdom of science."

The reports by Smith and other biographers who have published their studies concerning Pasteur's research notebooks after they were laid open (contrary to the desire of Pasteur that they never be opened) clearly support the contention that Pasteur frequently and conveniently forgot the work of predecessors and claimed their accomplishments as his own. What is even more astounding is that Pasteur knowingly and deliberately engaged in fraud in reporting results of his studies, especially in his work with vaccines.

John Waller in his detailed review of some of the "sins" of scientists characterized Pasteur as the most brilliant scientist who has ever lived, but also accused Pasteur of "making of very bold claims on the basis of less than comprehensive evidence. Pasteur was not above suppressing data that did not support his arguments against the spontaneous generation of life." What presumably prompted Kendall Smith's interest in the studies of vaccine developments by Pasteur was an experience he reported in his paper on medical immunology:

> I remembered that in 1998, while in France, I happened to read an article in Le Figaro, which announced that the anthrax vaccine introduced by Pasteur in 1881 was in fact not the live attenuated vaccine that Pasteur had suggested he used at the time. Instead, the vaccine was a chemically killed vaccine that had been developed and introduced by one of Pasteur's rivals, a Dr. Toussaint, who was a veterinarian from Toulouse, France.

To understand the implications of the announcement by a leading French newspaper that the icon of the French scientific accomplishment and integrity had committed what amounts to scientific fraud, it is necessary to research the source documents of Pasteur's experiments and publications.

Pasteur went on to claim that he had dispensed with the theory of "spontaneous generation," failing to mention any of the work performed by Lorenzo Spallanzani or Francesco Redi over one hundred years prior to Pasteur's curt announcement.

In 1878, Pasteur presented a report to the Academy of Sciences in France, outlining his studies of anthrax and claiming priority for the germ theory of disease.[8] Pasteur presented his studies on anthrax:

To demonstrate experimentally that a microscopic organism actually is the cause of a disease and the agent of contagion (anthrax), I know no other way, in the present state of Science, than to subject the microbe . . . to the method of cultivation out of the body. It may be noted that a culture serially diluted and cultivated a number of times in a sterile fluid medium would still retain the viability of producing anthrax in an animal. Such is—as we believe—the indisputable proof that anthrax is a bacterial disease.

It would appear that Pasteur was obsessed with the idea that air would be lethal to many microorganisms. He therefore, went on to address the Academy by indicating that:

It occurred to us that the septic vibrio might be an obligatory anaerobe and that the sterility of our inoculated culture fluids might be due to the destruction of the septic vibrio by the atmospheric oxygen dissolved in the fluids.

Results justified our attempt; the septic vibrio grew easily in a complete vacuum, and no less easily in the presence of pure carbonic acid. Furthermore all the vibrios, which crowded the liquid as motile threads, are destroyed and disappear. After the action of the air, only fine amorphous granules can be found unfit for culture as well as for the transmission of any disease whatever. It might be said that the air burned the vibrios.

. . . the effects of the anthrax bacteridium and the microbe of pus may be combined and the two diseases may be superposed, so as to obtain a purulent anthrax or an anthracoid purulent infection. Care must be taken not to exaggerate the predominance of the new microbe over the bacteridium. If the microbe be associated with the latter in sufficient amount, it may crowd it out completely— preventing it from growing in the body at all. Anthrax does not appear, and the infection, entirely local, becomes merely an abscess that is easy to cure. The microbe-producing pus and the septic vibrio (not)[9] being both anaerobes, as we have demonstrated, it is evident that the latter will not much disturb its neighbor.

Pasteur, with unabashed bluster, elected himself as the principal investigator proving the germ theory of disease:

> I asked the Academy not to dismiss these curious results before I demonstrate an important theoretical conclusion. We insist on demonstrating at the start of these studies (that are opening a whole new world of knowledge) a proof that the cause of transmissible, contagious and infectious diseases resides essentially and uniquely in the presence of microorganisms.

The report by Pasteur before the Academy on his experiments with the anthrax bacillus never even mentioned that Robert Koch had already demonstrated categorically that the culture of anthrax was the etiological agent of the disease. This demonstration took place two years before Pasteur went before the Academy claiming priority. Koch, the brilliant scientist that he was, not only carefully elaborated the criteria of confirming that an organism is the etiological agent of an infectious disease, but developed various cultural and staining techniques, which essentially are being used even to this day.

The colossal work of Agostino Bassi, which had been laid before the professional community and which earned him recognition by the French as well as many other governments, was passed over by Pasteur. Pasteur did not credit Bassi's achievements in postulating the germ theory of disease. Pasteur merely announced that his experiments demonstrated that all infectious diseases, such as smallpox, scarlet fever, rubella, syphilis, glanders, anthrax, yellow fever, typhus, and bovine plague, would be obliterated by preparing vaccines in the manner he had described for anthrax.

In Pasteur's presentation before the French Academy, he claimed that Edward Jenner's introduction of vaccination for smallpox about 100 years earlier was actually based on knowledge which had been known long before Jenner performed his work. It was Pasteur who then went on to claim the ability to effect immunity for all microbes, including smallpox, by his technology as evidence with the vaccine he had developed for anthrax.

Pasteur reported that his live attenuated vaccines, which were prepared by exposing them to air, were successful as vaccines for anthrax as well as for chicken cholera. When challenged to demonstrate the effectiveness of these vaccines, Pasteur agreed to a public demonstration utilizing his live atmospheric oxygen attenuated vaccine in protecting sheep. This public trial brought hundreds of observers, including a forum representing such varied professions as veterinarians, government officials, and local politicians.

However, only Pasteur and his collaborators presumably knew that the vaccine to be used for this trial was not a live attenuated vaccine prepared by exposing the organisms to air. Instead, the vaccine had been prepared by killing the organisms with a solution of potassium-bichromate, and was in fact, a vaccine composed of dead organisms and developed by the veterinarian Toussaint.

Despite the successful result of this vaccine by Pasteur, Robert Koch ultimately recognized the chicanery of Pasteur and became one of Pasteur's most outspoken critics. It is particularly puzzling how the self-styled genius of Pasteur was able to silence any criticism among those bacteriologists working in the late 19th century who knew that it was impossible to attenuate aerobic organisms by simply culturing them in the presence of air (Pasteur, 1863). The French government must have been aware of Pasteur's false claims through the complaints of Koch and Toussaint, who was the actual inventor of the vaccine against anthrax. Finally, in 1998, the French government was obliged to admit that the first successful vaccine against anthrax was developed by Toussaint.

Pasteur himself, as well as the French government and a number of his biographers, made a number of claims concerning his scientific achievements—some true and others at best highly exaggerated. For example, there were persistent reports (1) that Pasteur had developed concepts which introduced the science of immunology, (2) that Pasteur had disproved the validity of spontaneous generation, (3) that Pasteur's experiments with vaccines provided ubiquitous potential, (4) that he was the preeminent pioneer in introducing the concept of the germ theory of disease, (5) that Pasteur had developed concepts which led to the use of pasteurization of milk and other nutritive fluids, and (6) that his development of looped appendages of flasks supported his refutation of the theory of spontaneous generation. These and other musings by Pasteur's biographers led to the belief that Pasteur was a great scientist and humanitarian.

In a paper published in the American Society for Microbiology News, James E. Strick points out that one attribute of the genius of Pasteur was not permitting himself to be too rigidly bound by concepts. Thus, Pasteur had taken the position that parasitic worms could arise by spontaneous generation, and this position had been essentially concealed in his notes and was not discovered until about 1917. Thus, he kept silent about his own experiments to support the concept of spontaneous generation while publicly refuting the work of Pouchet, who was an advocate of the theory of spontaneous generation. Pasteur claimed, as have some of his biographers, that he never filed any patents for his inventions. Instead, he maintained, he offered them freely to all that would use them for the sake of humanity. Merely a superficial examination of the records of various patent offices (Federico, 1937) indicates that Pasteur filed patents in France, Italy, and the United States. At the last count approximately 35 patents were filed by him in his name.

Pasteur died on September 28, 1895, and the position of head of the Pasteur Institute was assumed by Eli Metchnikoff. Metchnikoff, together with Paul Ehrlich, was credited with performing the pioneer studies that made possible the concepts of immunology and the methods by which vaccines could be utilized to protect against infectious disease.

NOTES

1. The biographer Debré provides a very detailed understanding of the origin and ancestors of Pasteur, his education, and the influence that his parents had on his education.

2. The documented revelations by Ethel Douglas Hume and others have begun to prompt statements, such as those by Mary Bellis, that "A few historians disagree with the accepted wisdom regarding Pasteur and believe that the evidence points to him as being a plagiarizer and fraud of note, and that his research was not at all original. The following Web sites support this view: *The Myth of Pasteurization, Pasteur also a Faker: Antisepsis,* and *The Private Science of Louis Pasteur.*

3. Scholars are generally in uniform agreement that Redi, working approximately 200 years before Pasteur, had performed conclusive experiments refuting the concept of spontaneous generation.

4. In 1885 Amiel Christian Hanson working at the Carlsberg Laboratory established for the first time the use of pure yeast cultures to be used in the fermentation of beer, thus significantly improving our understanding of the fermentation process.

5. From the Statutes of the State of Minnesota regulating the bacteria counts of milk. Coliform organisms present in milk invariably result from fecal contamination.

6. The biography by Geison (1995) was essentially the first volume which reported in detail the activities of Pasteur, which led the author to indicate that Pasteur practiced numerous outright deceptions in order to establish his position, to fund his laboratory, and to massage his ego. (Geison's biography of Pasteur was reviewed by Brock, 1995.)

7. With the opening of the research books of Louis Pasteur, contrary to Pasteur's wishes, concerning the experiments and the details provided by Pasteur's research efforts on page 108 of his research notebook, it is now possible to assess the priority of the claims of Pasteur for his studies with the swan-necked flasks.

8. Pasteur, L. *et al.*, 1878.

9. The translator felt that Pasteur had made a mistake in characterizing both organisms as anaerobes and has arbitrarily corrected the 'mistake' by adding the word (not) in order to correct the error.

Chapter Ten

Charles Chamberland

Long before anyone was able to characterize the role of infectious bacteria in water, many people realized that water could act as a source of certain diseases. Hippocrates, considered the father of modern medicine, recommended that rainwater should be routinely boiled and strained in order to remove odiferous agents from the water which otherwise would cause hoarseness. Aristotle, the Greek philosopher, is reputed to have advised Alexander the Great to have his soldiers not drink from stagnant pools, but to carry only boiled water on their expeditions. The filtration of water to remove particulate matter and effect a certain degree of clarity so that standing water may be drunk was instituted as early as 1832 in Richmond, Virginia. The city installed sand beds through which water was permitted to pass. Such filtration beds strained out a considerable amount of the suspended particles and, in part, some disease organisms. Filtration beds at that time consisted of various types of filtration media, such as crushed coal or sand. Various methods of filtration were tested and patented, but essentially all operated under the same principle of slowly passing water through filter beds.

It was primarily to these problems of effecting a safe mechanism for clarifying water that one of Pasteur's young colleagues, Charles Chamberland, began to experiment with unglazed porcelain. Water would slowly flow through the porcelain, especially under a small amount of pressure. At the same time, the essentially microscopic porosity of the unglazed porcelain could keep out suspended particles in the water as well as microorganisms. But it was not known at that time, because of the lack of technical equipment, that even the unglazed porcelain could not remove viruses.

Chamberland was born in Chilly-le-Vignoble, France, in 1851. He concentrated in mathematics at college in Paris and in 1871 was admitted to the

École Normale Superior, where his studies were concentrated in the physical sciences. From 1875 to 1879, he served as a laboratory attendant to Pasteur at the École Normale Superior in Paris. Pasteur soon recognized the superior innovations and intellect of Chamberland and in 1879, he named Chamberland his laboratory director.

Chamberland's education in physics bore fruit when he conceived of a superior method of sterilization. In this method, the pressure in a chamber could be increased by generating steam at a higher than atmospheric pressure, thus resulting in a temperature high enough to kill all living microorganisms. This method of sterilization was characterized as an *autoclave* and has been utilized by laboratories throughout the world to sterilize equipment. Medical products that could be sterilized in an autoclave had to be able to withstand a pressure of approximately 15 pounds per square inch and a temperature with steam that would reach 120–140° C. The Chamberland autoclave became one of the principal mechanisms of sterilization in hospitals throughout the world. The autoclave, invented by Chamberland, also became a ubiquitous tool in sterilizing canned goods, which then could be maintained in the sterile sealed state for years without deterioration. Based on Chamberland's work, home pressure cookers became a household utensil for quickly cooking foods.

In 1884, experimenting with unglazed porcelain, Chamberland developed a filter through which bacteriological cultures, water, and other fluids could be passed. All particulate matter and bacteria could be trapped and removed, resulting in an effluent which only contained viruses and biological biochemicals in solution. Pasteur quickly recognized the important application of such a device, not only for laboratory use, but for the purification of contaminated water. He quickly acted to file appropriate patents and set up companies that would manufacture the Chamberland filter, to which he affixed his name as the Pasteur-Chamberland filter.

The Chamberland filter made it possible to separate out the debris from bacteriological cultures and procure a purified effluent that would pass through the filter. The filter would permit only very small molecules and viruses to pass, but it would present an impasse to all particulate matter.

In the development of many communities in the United States, it was early recognized that drinking water would have to be treated in order to remove insoluble debris and any particulate matter that could be deleterious to the population drinking such water. An early attempt to provide such clarified water took place in 1832 in Richmond, Virginia, as described earlier. It was recognized as early as 1887 that the introduction of sand beds to filter drinking water for a city would remove not only particulate matter, but even infectious organisms such as cholera and typhoid.

A historical review of the water system of Philadelphia cited the important role that the Pasteur-Chamberland Filter Company was playing in purifying the water of the Schuylkill River:

> Due to the Pasteur-Chamberland Filter Company in 1890,[1] the Philadelphia water troubles are at an end. The Schuylkill River water made pure, healthful and clear as crystal, and free from all germs of typhoid fever, cholera, cholera infantum, diphtheria, etc., by being purified through the only germproof filter in the world—the Pasteur germ-proof water filter. . . .

Companies were set up by investors to capitalize on the application of such filters for the purification of water. One such company was established in Dayton, Ohio, and one of its advertisements was released circa 1889.

The following is from a pamphlet advertising this firm's water filter. At the time, Philadelphia's water was infamous for its poor quality. It did indeed carry typhoid and other diseases. A World War I era cartoon even alleged that "fighting the Kaiser" would be safer than staying home and drinking the water:

> The Pasteur-Chamberland Filter Company
> 61 South Wyandot Street, Dayton, Ohio
>
> It is now removed beyond per adventure of doubt, that very many of the diseases of man may be traced to impure water used for drinking purposes, and it is curious to observe the indifference of many, who without a thought, daily and hourly absorb poison in their system when, with but little expense and scarcely any trouble, they could free the water they drink from all deleterious, organic or poisonous matter. The Pasteur-Chamberland Filter Co., of this city, are making a filter which entirely performs all that is claimed for it, and that is the absolute purifying of water from every particle of deleterious matter, no matter how minute if held in suspension. The company was incorporated in December 1887, and they are the sole licenses for the manufacture of the Pasteur filters in the United States, Canada, and Mexico. About five years ago, Pasteur, the celebrated French scientist, in conjunction with Mr. Charles E. Chamberland, began to devote his attention to the discovery of a medium of filtration which would render water and other fluids absolutely free from germs of all kind and other organic matter, as pure water was imperative to him in his researches for the discovery of the germs which produced certain diseases, notably hydrophobia and phylloxera. The result, after ten years of experiment, was the celebrated Pasteur Filter. This was in 1884 and M. Pasteur said of it, "knowing its full scientific and hygienic value I desire it to bear my name," and the reputation of this eminent man is such that anything thus endowed by him cannot but be of superlative merit.
>
> By the use of these filters we are exempted from drinking muddy, polluted and warm water, and all risk of contracting typhoid fever, diphtheria, dysentery

and other zymotic diseases is entirely obviated. From the faucet of the Pasteur Perfection Filter and Cooler flows forth a stream of pure, sparkling and cool water, free from all germs of disease, and all organic matter held in suspension. The principal of these filters is entirely different from all others and neither sand, gravel, charcoal nor alum are used as filtering mediums. These materials do not take out any germs or finer organisms which really hold the poison, on the contrary they often concentrate them in one place. The Pasteur Filter is constructed upon an entirely distant plan. It consists of one or more hollow porcelain tubes which in appearance resemble a candle having no opening, except for an orifice at one end through which the purified water is discharged. No impurities whatever penetrate this material but are arrested on the outside where they can be readily removed. These tubes all come from France, where alone the material is found of which they are made. They can be easily cleaned as an ordinary lamp chimney. The company publishes a neat little illustrated pamphlet which fully explains the merits of these appliances, and they will cheerfully forward the same upon application as well as all other particulars.

The filters are made in a number of sizes and designs, and they are very attractive and handsome in appearance. They have received the endorsement of scientists, physicians and others all over this country and Europe, and made at the works in Dayton and the factory consists of a three story brick building, 70×110 feet in dimensions, equipped throughout with new machinery and appliances.

The President of the company is Mr. A.A. Blount, Mr. T.S. Babbit is Vice President, and Mr. J. S. Miles, Secretary and General Manager. Conducting an enterprise of a most useful and progressive character, the Pasteur-Chamberlain Filter Co. is entitled to the utmost consideration, and apart from a business standpoint, are doing much good in producing an appliance which combats to a large extent the ravages of fell disease, and provides a safeguard otherwise difficult if not impossible to obtain elsewhere.

In August of 1898, the Pasteur Chamberland Filter Co. was destroyed by fire. Loss was $20,000. The cause was unknown.

The early Chamberland filters prepared from unglazed porcelain had pores that were significantly smaller than the size of bacteria or approximately 0.1 micrometer. Since it was thus possible to pass a solution that contained bacteria through one of these Chamberland filters, the medium that passed through and was therefore free of all bacteria was considered sterile. Such sterility, having been achieved without the use of heat, ultimately became a procedure for the removal of bacteria from various solutions. Suppose that a diseased animal or man provided blood serum or a specimen from a lesion that, when inoculated into a healthy animal, would cause disease. It could be concluded that the disease was transmitted by bacteria if the same specimen from an infected animal or person was passed through a Chamberland filter and did not cause the disease. Thus, the evidence would be more apparent that the bacteria were the causative agent of the disease transmitted without the use of the filtrate through the Chamberland filter.

Subsequent studies, however, of diseases such as that caused by the tobacco mosaic virus resulted in the conclusion that there were invisible microorganisms which caused the disease. In studies conducted by Adolf Mayer, he was able to show that injecting fluid extracts from a diseased, discolored tobacco plant into a healthy plant would transmit the tobacco mosaic disease to the healthy plant. When the extracts were passed through a Chamberland filter before being injected into a healthy plant, they still caused the disease, even though no bacteria passed through the Chamberland filter. The early conclusions were that the filter might have been cracked, or that there might be causative agents that could pass through the filter and transmit the disease.

It was not until 1898 when the Dutch botanist Martinus Beijerinck, continuing these experiments with tobacco mosaic disease, came to the conclusion that the disease agent must be much smaller than bacteria. Not being able to see or identify it, he called the organism a living fluid (*contagium vivum fluidum*). The initial conclusions of Beijerinck and others working with the tobacco mosaic disease postulated that these filterable solutions, free of bacteria, could contain a toxin which resulted in the disease; or because serially transferring the filtrate from a diseased plant to healthy plants still resulted in the tobacco mosaic infection, which was characterized by these light-green and dark-green areas on the plant. Consequently, it was concluded that a toxin could not be the etiological agent, because a toxin would be diluted out by serial transfer; and therefore, it probably was due to a living organism that was too small to be a bacterium. The term for these ultra-filtrable particles was coined, referring to them as *viruses,* which in Latin means *poison*.

Chamberland went on to develop significant improvements in his filters. Consequently, such improvements in the filters were filed as patents by Chamberland in a British Patent Office in 1900, namely British Patent Number 7283, and again in 1901, under British Patent Number 25,606; in the British Patent Office in 1904 under British Patent Number 27,180, and in 1911 in the British Patent Office under Patent Number 16,270.

By 1911, Chamberland had considerably enlarged the scope of materials out of which these filtering apparatuses could be manufactured, including porcelain, asbestos, charcoal, and cellulose. Asbestos pad filters continued in use into the 1940's, and charcoal filters are still in use for specific applications. Typical drawings showing the construction of Chamberland's filters are depicted from his 1904 patent and reproduced here in Figure 10.1.

Chamberland for a number of years continued to improve his filtration apparatus. Patents, especially in the United Kingdom, were issued in 1902,

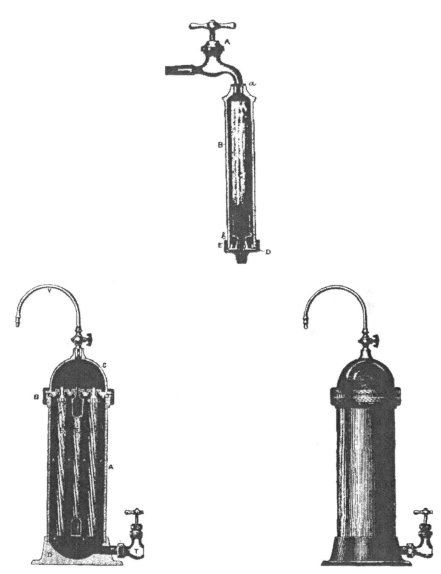

Figure 10.1. Filters designed by Charles Chamberland.

1905, and 1911. The development of the Chamberland filter ultimately led to the discovery of viruses because the filters could not remove viruses.

In the early 1900's, the French-Canadian microbiologist Félix d'Herelle discovered a virus that infected and killed bacteria. He had inoculated bacteria into Petri dishes in order to permit them to grow. Frequently an opaque growth of bacteria appeared across the plate, but periodically he observed clear round spots, which did not contain any growth of the bacteria. In his researches, D'Herelle, using a fine needle, picked up a small amount of the surface of the clear area on the plate and transferred it to an area of the plate where the bacteria had grown in a confluent manner. Then, after incubation, he observed that portions of the area which originally contained bacteria now presumably had dissolved, leaving a clear space. Observations under the microscope yielded nothing out of the ordinary. Taking a bacterial culture and passing it through a Chamberland filter removed all of the bacteria, but the clear liquid still retained the ability, when placed on an inoculated plate, to dissolve the bacteria, resulting in clear round spots on the plate.

This led D'Herelle to believe that whatever was dissolving the bacteria must be far smaller than bacteria, and just beyond the capability of the microscopes available at that time to make them visible. D'Herelle's experiments in which a liquid culture of bacteria was permitted to grow resulted in a cloudy growth of organisms. If he picked up one of the clear spots on an inoculated plate with a sterile needle and transferred the contents of the needle into a culture of cloudy organisms, following incubation, the medium would again appear to be clear. Again, this indicated that something too small to be detected was killing the bacteria. Observations under the microscope during the period when bacteria were gradually dying were able to show D'Herelle that the bacterial organisms would begin to swell, and ultimately the organisms would disappear by becoming completely dissolved. D'Herelle named these invisible particles that passed through a Chamberland filter *bacteriophages*.

A few decades earlier, Pasteur and Chamberland performed similar experiments revealing that blood from a rabid dog would show no living bacteria. However, it would contain something that would pass through a Chamberland filter and, when inoculated into a healthy animal, would ultimately cause rabies. At first, it was thought that these small particles were minute bacteria that were beyond the view of the microscopes available at the time, or they could be some protein particle that would have the ability to kill bacteria and cause disease. A common criterion for any organism being characterized as "living" is the ability to have autonomous metabolic activity if permitted to grow in a suitable environment; the viruses do not exhibit any autonomous metabolic activity and, therefore, cannot be characterized as having "life."

The demonstration by D'Herelle that there existed such ultra-microscopic and filterable particles that could kill living cells, albeit bacteria, opened up the vista for the examination of many other diseases—including smallpox, yellow fever, the mosaic disease of tobacco plants, and poliomyelitis—all of which have been shown since these early studies to be caused by viruses.

It would be some time after the discoveries of D'Herelle that microbiologists would begin to consider the possibility that certain viruses might be used therapeutically—that is, they would be highly specific in killing pathogenic microorganisms if it could be shown that the viruses in and of themselves were not harmful to humans.

Although scientists concluded that viruses themselves have no metabolic activity and therefore cannot be considered "living," they found that viruses can survive and multiply in the presence of susceptible cells. They learned that a number of viruses can even be crystallized—and can be confused with ordinary table salt—and still retain their ability to cause disease when reintroduced into a susceptible host.

Subsequent inventions by Chamberland did achieve a filter that would filter out viruses. Although the ultimate goal of filtration was to remove all particulate matter including viruses, there were useful purposes to be served by using the early so-called Chamberland filters which permitted viruses to pass through their porosity. In 1919 a veterinarian, J.S. Koen, observed that pigs had a disease which resembled the human influenza of the 1918 epidemic. This observation was later confirmed by Richard Schoep working at the Rockefeller Institute of Comparative Anatomy. Schoep (1919) obtained extracts from sick pigs and passed them through a Chamberland filter. He found that the viruses contained in the filtrate would reproduce the disease when injected into healthy pigs, thus providing evidence of the viral transmission of the so-called pig influenza from one animal to another.

Having been made aware by Pasteur that he desired to extrapolate his studies on the pathology of the silkworm to animal and human diseases, Chamberland approached Pasteur in the spring of 1887 and suggested the possibility of bringing in a research worker who had been concerned with observations concerning the immunology of the disease process. Approaching Pasteur, Chamberland said, "I have seen a number of reports regarding a publication by a zoologist who discovered that resistance to certain bacteria might be explained by the presence of certain white blood cells which literally engulf the bacteria so destroying them and protect the infected animal from infection and disease."

Pasteur: "What do you know about this person?"

Chamberland: "He is a Russian who has been a professor in zoology and comparative anatomy at the University of Odessa, and subsequently worked in a private laboratory and reported his observations which he had characterized as phagocytosis."

Pasteur: "Are you sure that this is a valid observation? I don't recall that any of us had ever seen such a phenomenon during our studies where any animal or human cells would swallow up bacteria and so destroy them."

Chamberland: "These studies of Metchnikoff have been confirmed by a number of other research workers. It has been reported in the Compt. Rend.

Académie des sciences of Paris in an article by Balbiani that crickets cannot be infected with large numbers of bacteria of the group *Bacillus subtilis*. He confirmed the observations that the white blood cells of pericardial tissue which corresponds to certain elements of the spleen were engulfing these organisms.

"Furthermore, insects such as butterflies, flies, and other insects have very few white blood cells or leucocytes as they call them, and are found to be susceptible to infection with the same bacteria. This would tend to indicate a relationship between the immunity to these bacteria and the presence of this destruction by white blood cells."

Pasteur countered with: "Why don't we wait until we see how our work progresses before we call in a foreigner to join our group?" With this final statement, Pasteur left the room.

By the spring of 1888, Pasteur was convinced that they did, in fact, require someone trained and working in the field of immunology. Pasteur finally conceded and instructed Chamberland to invite Elie Metchnikoff to join their group at the Institute.

NOTE

1. The early history of the water system of Philadelphia is from the collective data of Dr. Murphy, University of Pennsylvania, 1975.

Chapter Eleven

Bassi—Coda

Agostino Bassi is considered the founder of the parasitic theory of infectious disease. In his honor, a postage stamp, Figure 11.1, was issued on September 5, 1953, to coincide with the 6th International Congress of Microbiology held in Rome.

The portrait of Bassi on the stamp is draped with the life cycle of the silkworm, the studies of which launched Bassi's research which accorded him the distinction of being considered the founder and principal proponent of the parasitic theory of infectious diseases.

Problems of infectious diseases are as real and urgent in the 21st century as they were nearly a thousand years ago. Such diseases still decimate large numbers of the population and challenge medical researchers to determine the causes of these infections and methods by which they can be prevented or treated. Because we now know that microorganisms may mutate and become resistant to therapeutic measures or become more virulent, and because the populations of the earth have increased and created overcrowding—especially in the world's largest cities—the problems that face us today in achieving protection against infections are probably far more taxing than ever before. David Morens, Gregory Folkers, and Anthony Fauci in an excellent review of emerging infections (2008) have characterized some of the examples of epidemics that occurred from 430 B.C. to the 20th century and the vast numbers of populations that were decimated by such infections as indicated by Table 11.1.

The Black Death of the 1340's, which killed about 50 million people, was far more devastating than the Spanish influenza of 1918, which also decimated approximately 50 million, because the world population was far less in the 1340's than it was in 1918.

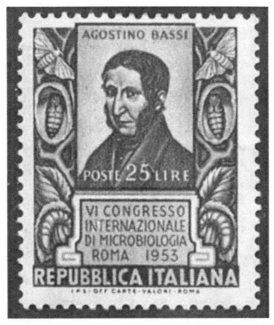

Figure 11.1.   The postage stamp issued by the Italian government honoring Bassi.

Table 11.1.   Examples of Epidemic Emerging Infections of Historical Interest from Morens et al., 2008

Period of Time	Emerging Disease	Causal Agent	Estimated Number of Human Deaths
430-426 BCE	Plague of Athens	Unidentified	40,000
1340s	Black Death	*Yersinia pestis*	50 million
1494–99	French pox (syphilis)	*Treponema pallidum*	>50,000
1520–21	*Hueyzahuatl* (smallpox)	Variola major	3.5 million
1700s	European cattle Epizootics	Rinderpest virus, foot and mouth disease virus, *Bacillus anthracis*	>15,000*
1793–98	The American plague	Yellow fever virus	25,000
1832	2nd cholera pandemic, Paris	*Vibrio chloerae*	18,402
1875	Fiji virgin soil epidemic	Measles virus	40,000
1918–19	Spanish influenza	H1N1 influenza virus	≥50 million
From 1981	AIDS pandemic	HIV	>25 million

*The deaths referred to in the 1700s refers to cattle deaths, instead of human deaths.

The methods and technology available today for detecting infectious diseases and studying mechanisms—and thus preventing or treating them—are certainly much more advanced than what was available to Agostino Bassi when he undertook his studies of the silkworm disease. The elucidating and characterizing of the studies of Bassi are intended not only to understand the silkworm disease, but also to understand the role that infectious organisms play in acting as the agents for many other diseases which were prevalent and studied at his time. The intention is also to give credit to Bassi as one of the first persons to understand and to postulate the infectious nature of diseases. Such credit is particularly cogent for a person who professionally began his career as an attorney and suffered bouts of blindness, which oftentimes curtailed his work at the microscope and restricted his ability to continue his studies. In addition, we have found no patents that Bassi chose to procure for himself.

On January 12, 1923, the Medical-Surgical Society of Pavia marked the one-hundredth anniversary of the birth of Louis Pasteur (born December 27, 1822). Besides honoring Pasteur, the Society concomitantly honored the works of Agostino Bassi. The principal address was made by Camillo Golgi, a renowned scientist in his own right. The discussions and presentations at this meeting were ultimately published in 1925 under the auspices of the Societa Medico-Chirurgica Di Pavia. The salient aspects that were elaborated are as follows:

> Despite the fact that Bassi had been educated as a lawyer, he was able to acquire and capitalize on the teachings of Spallanzani to which he was more inclined than to practice law. By his pursuits in exploring the fundamentals of modern pathogenesis of infectious diseases and utilizing a methodical plan of observations and experiments carefully laid out and patiently followed over a long period of time, he not only was able to discover the pathogenesis of the silkworm disease, but was able to continue and elaborate by analogy and generalization of proven facts, the germ theory of disease. The germ theory was decidedly affirmed by him for many contagious diseases both for man and animals.
>
> Silk was one of the major products, not only of our kingdom, but for all of Italy. Therefore, it is very important to know how to raise the precious animals properly. A lot has been written on this topic, especially by Count Vincenzo Dandolo, but until now, nobody, not in Italy, nor in France, or anybody else, has been able to prevent the terrible massacre that the disease we call *Calcinetto,* and the French call muscardine, causes among the silkworms. Doctor Bassi observed and studied the situation for over 20 years and his incredible observations continued with diversified experiments, great labor, and fatigue, finally came to the conclusion that he had discovered the true nature of the deadly disease and also the means to prevent it and the means to extirpate it once it is manifested.

He was very glad to have made such a precious discovery since at the time, because of the things that had happened to him, he did not have much money and he had a lot of need. So he kept some of his findings secret, hoping, not without a reason, to be able to obtain by means of it not only enough for his needs, but perhaps to establish an income. He decided on inviting the princes, agricultural societies, scientific societies, and rich landowners to buy his precious findings. But since his assertions were not generally accepted, and since so many people had spent so much time studying, meditating, and making experiments on such a topic, and these were very well known agriculturalists from Italy and abroad, nobody asked about his findings. It took several years before Bassi's discoveries could be useful to silkworm raisers. Although Bassi tried to keep it a secret because it was such an important discovery, he ultimately decided that public good had to go before his own good, so he made his discovery public.

In 1835 Bassi published his research concerning the disease of silkworms entitled *Del mal del segno, calcinaccio o moscardino, malattia che affligge I bachi da sela esulmodo di liberarne le bigattaie anche le più infestate.*

This report was concerned with the theoretical aspects of the disease which he had shown to be caused by a fungus. The fungus originally had been characterized as *Beauveria*, but later was renamed *Beauveria bassiana* in honor of Bassi.

A year later, in 1836, Bassi outlined the practical considerations of caring for the silkworm to reduce the risk of infection with the mold. The monographs published by Bassi in 1836 and a subsequent addition published in 1837 characterized the conclusions that Bassi had made following his many years of study. Bassi had demonstrated that:

1. Preventative measures for the silkworm disease would require that silkworm eggs should be disinfected with dilute solutions of calcium chloride, alcohols, or nitric acid.
2. When eggs were purchased from outside sources, the containers for these eggs should be disinfected or destroyed by burning.
3. Fresh uncontaminated mulberry leaves must be used for feeding the healthy silkworms.
4. Instruments and any appliances used in the nursery raising the silkworms should be disinfected in boiling water or exposed to fire.
5. The crowded conditions where the silkworms were raised should be avoided.
6. All workers entering the facility where the silkworms were raised should practice hygienic measures. They should wear protective clothing that could be boiled or otherwise washed in solutions that would decontaminate infected clothing. In addition, workers should always wash their hands after having contact with any diseased silkworms.

These measures for preventing the infection of healthy organisms by infectious agents that had invaded diseased silkworms were very revolutionary in Bassi's time and, in fact, did not result in uniform acceptance. Bassi's subsequent studies also showed that the same criteria he had set forth in the prevention of cross-infection from infected silkworms or infected mulberry leaves could be extrapolated to other disease organisms. Thus the idea of disinfection of instruments, tables, trays, and clothing that is used in any facility where infectious organisms were prevalent gradually won acceptance and was implemented on a world-wide basis albeit many years after Bassi's initial experiments had elucidated this criteria.[1]

These publications for the first time elaborated research reports of Bassi in which he had demonstrated:

1. That the disease of silkworm was caused by a microorganism; and that this microorganism, when taken from an infected silkworm, would transmit the disease to an uninfected silkworm.
2. Extrapolating from these diseases of silkworms and other disease organisms, which have been reported in man and animals, Bassi concluded for the first time that infectious diseases in man and animals were caused by microorganisms.
3. Bassi's experiments demonstrated that the etiological agent of an infectious disease could be demonstrated by isolating an organism from an infected host, which when transmitted to a healthy animal or man would cause the same disease. They further demonstrated that these infectious organisms could be cultivated outside of the body of the infected animal or man and when inoculated back into a healthy animal would cause the same disease.
4. Not only did Bassi freely reveal his methodology for the detection of silkworm fungus disease, but he also freely revealed the chemicals he had used to disinfect the areas and to wash one's hands, and the application of incineration. These procedures have achieved ubiquitous applications in health care facilities in practically all nations of the world.

These attributes of infection were later repeated and characterized almost exactly as Bassi had characterized them by the brilliant Robert Koch, after which they came to be known as Koch's postulates.

Bassi's studies and reports concerning his experiments with the silkworms were attributed to rescuing the important silk industry in Italy, and ultimately in other countries that adopted Bassi's experimental methods. These reports, translated into French and distributed throughout Europe, brought immediate fame to Bassi. Meanwhile, Bassi continued to expand his concepts of the

germ theory of disease, explaining how plants and animals—including human beings—were susceptible to pathogenic organisms. Bassi claimed that
his research efforts indicated microorganisms were the etiological agents of
infectious diseases. In his book, he wrote: "I would be very happy if in the
future, my discoveries served to open up study and find cures for the fatal
diseases which affect mankind, including cholera."

In 1953, on the 180th anniversary of Bassi's birth in 1773, and in conjunc-
tion with an international conclave of microbiologists meeting in Rome at
that time, the Italian government issued a stamp honoring Agostino Bassi.
The stamp featured a portrait of Bassi bordered by sketches of silkworms in
both pupa and adult stages.

Landowners, agriculturists, people who loved the public good, and a number of agricultural and scientific academies gave the inventor much praise
and thanks. He became a member of the Society of Sciences and Crafts of
Italy and also of France and of Germany. He was nominated a member of the
Royal Institute of Sciences, Literature, and Art in Milan. He was awarded a
gold medal from the Archduke of Rainieri and another gold medal from the
emperor of Austria with a declaration for civil merit of 2nd Class of Austria,
and also a sum of a thousand fiorini. When Count Giacomo Barbo of Milan
went to Paris, after the important discoveries of Bassi had been published in
Italian, Bassi's two volumes of *The Theory* and *Practice* on Conchino were
also published in French. The king of France was very grateful to Doctor
Bassi. He gave Bassi a gold medal and he gave Count Barbo a silver medal.
Later on, the same king showed even more gratitude to Bassi by making him
a Knight of the Royal Order of the Legion of Honor of France.

Bassi later gave the Royal Scientific Institute in Paris some memoirs on
his research. The abovementioned work by Bassi on conchino, also called
the disease of sine, does not include only the method to prevent the deadly
disease and to extirpate it once it is shown in the silkworm. It also includes
Bassi's discovery of a better way of raising silkworms so that every possible
advantage can be gotten from them.

But it would be of very little help to know the good way of raising silkworms if one did not know the best way of growing the plant from which
they get their necessary nutrition. This work, which we know as the cultivation of mulberries, is no doubt the one by Count Carlo Verri, but Bassi felt
that Verri's document had a number of mistakes. It does not teach the best
way of cultivating mulberries, and it also has obscure points. Bassi, after a
long series of comparative experiments, and after many years of practice and
studies in the field with his own mulberry trees, determined the best way of
growing this plant in nature.

A contemporary of Bassi wrote that: Bassi's research would be published soon, correcting mistakes that existed in Verri's treatise. Bassi felt that it was generally understood that agriculture in Lodi was the best of all in Italy and perhaps the best of all in Europe. Until then, nobody had published work on it. This perhaps was due, in small part, to the well-known professor, Doctor Bassi, who has described it at length. It came to light in a publication entitled *Agricultural Practice as It is Reasoned in the Lodi Province.*

Although the elaboration by Bassi of the germ theory of disease was primarily based on his studies with silkworms, his efforts extended to other avenues of research, which further opened the door to investigation by other scientists. Thus, Bassi investigated the cultivation of potatoes and published a treatise on that topic. He published a treatise on the raising of sheep. He studied wine production from various fruits, such as cherries and oranges. Bassi also studied the preparation of cheeses—more particularly the famous cheeses of Lodi—and wrote a report on these studies in 1820.

Unfortunately, Bassi gradually became blind. As a result, his work, especially that involving microscopy, was so impaired that his research became relatively forgotten. However, a number of scholars continued to follow his studies.

As a result of the research by Bassi, we now have his well-documented discoveries of the causes of contagious diseases, which were elaborated at a time when we were still very far from the contemporary scientific views. Bassi was able to predict and affirm principles that today are some of the strongholds of our conceptions of parasitic disease:

1. In every case where the silkworms are shown to be infected, the disease organisms could be found, isolated, and identified.
2. The transfer of the infectious organisms from silkworm larvae so infected, when transmitted to healthy silkworms, would cause the same disease as that described in the original infected silkworm larvae from which the organisms were isolated.

It was fortunate that Bassi's interests in science moved him from the practice of law into fields of study that had their beginning in the transition from natural philosophy to biological research.

Italy had enjoyed an unparalleled status in the field of science until the beginning of the 19th century. At that time, major political developments diverted attention from the sciences. Giuseppi Garibaldi's efforts contributed to a treaty where the various states of Italy would combine to form the nation of Italy. Emphasis in the biological and medical sciences began to shift from Italy to other countries, where distinguished scientists and researchers were performing studies that would alter the knowledge and practice of medicine, chemistry, and microbiology. One of the most distinguished scientists was the German, Robert Koch, whose studies of tuberculosis and other infectious diseases resulted in the postulates, known to this day as "Koch's postulates." These postulates were almost identical to the postulates of Bassi, which were enumerated in the 1850's as the criteria by which one could determine what disease could be identified as being microbial in origin.

Following Bassi's publications and public announcements, a wave of research predicated on Bassi's concepts of the germ theory of disease began to occur. The role of Bassi and his work which was the initial series of investigations that documented the infectious nature of disease was not overlooked by everyone, certainly not by many members of the scientific community. However, because of the tremendous acclaim that Pasteur was able to engender, many of the reports that preceded Pasteur were fortuitously or conveniently overlooked.

Bassi's discovery of the organism that is the etiological agent for the silkworm disease, renamed in his honor as *Beauveria bassiana,* was followed soon after by the discovery of a number of human diseases caused by fungi, such as the etiological agents for candidiasis, aspergillosis, and blastomycosis. Despite the ubiquitous nature of some of these diseases, the more devastating diseases at that time were those caused by microorganisms, such as those of the bubonic plague, pneumonia, syphilis, and tuberculosis. A paper published by Renata Rivera Ferreira and Robert de Andrade Martins (1997) succinctly cited Bassi's research as being the first case which showed conclusively and experimentally the causal relationship between microorganisms and disease.

The mystique of the cause and etiology of infections in man and animal had now been broken and there followed an avalanche of research and investigation. The publications by Bassi encouraged studies by other investigators. Two years after Bassi's reports were published, Robert Remak observed the presence of fungal growth in men infected on the scalp. The causative agents were later identified as molds causing *tinea favus*. Remak was probably the first person to demonstrate that a human infection was caused by a fungus microorganism.

In an article by Conte Giacomo (Jacques) Barbò,[2] published in 1836, the discourse of Bassi's studies for muscardine was reviewed in detail. Barbò described the various forms of the silkworm in the healthy state and when infected with muscardine as reported by Bassi and as shown in Figure 11.2.

Johann Schoenlein, a German medical researcher and professor, lauded Bassi's work in an introduction, *Zur Pathogenie der Impetigines.*[3]

A little later in 1841, David Grub isolated a mold from a skin infection in a human and showed that this fungus could cause ringworm when inoculated into normal skin.

In 1845, Miles Berkeley was able to identify the fungus that was responsible for the potato blight in Ireland and it was named *Phytopthora infestans*.

In 1846, Ignace Semmelweis, a Hungarian obstetrician and professor at the University of Vienna, succeeded in reducing the mortality in the maternity ward from 27 percent to 0.23 percent simply by requiring that midwives and doctors charged with the examination of patients wash their hands with a solution of bleach. Despite the fact that the reduction in mortality of patients was impressive, many of the doctors at that time resisted the suggestions of Semmelweis. Such resistance may have contributed to his psychiatric problems. Semmelweis became insane and died of an infection following a cut on his hand made during a dissection of a cadaver.

Robert Koch can be regarded as one of the principal developers of the science of microbiology. It was he who developed many laboratory methods still in use today, including nutritive media adapted to different species of bacteria and the culturing of bacteria on solid media. One owes him thanks for, among other things, the discovery of the bacillus of tuberculosis and the vibrio of cholera.

In 1894, Japanese researchers discovered and identified the *bacillus* of plague, which had devastated so many parts of Europe in the Middle Ages. They also discovered the disease organism for dysentery in 1897.

Patrick Manson, an English researcher in tropical medicine, reported in 1877 that insects could carry the embryos of the organism which causes elephantiasis (filariasis). He later determined that this organism is transmitted by a mosquito. In 1881 Carlos Finlay, working in Cuba, was able to show that yellow fever was carried by a mosquito. Based largely on these studies, Walter Reed and William Crawford Gorgas were able to reduce the incidence of yellow fever among American workers building the Panama Canal.

During Bassi's silkworm studies, he pursued investigations to determine if any antiseptic procedures could be utilized to kill the organisms that caused the disease in the silkworm. Included among the techniques Bassi recommended was the clean and aseptic handling of the silkworms to ensure that there would be no contamination from silkworms that may have been infected with parasitic fungi. Bassi recommended the use of disinfectants such as calcium chloride to disinfect areas where the silkworm was growing and to ensure the destruction of the fungal growth that was so devastating to colonies of the silkworm.

These studies were very encouraging to those physicians that worked in hospitals where infectious diseases, without the use of antiseptic methods, were responsible for a very high percentage of deaths, especially those fol-

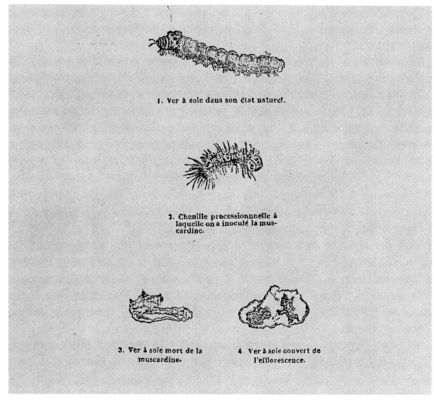

1. Ver à soie daus son état naturel.

2. Chenille processionnnelle à laquelle on a inoculé la muscardine.

3. Ver à soie mort de la muscardine.

4. Ver à soie couvert de l'efflorescence.

Figure 11.2.   Description of the organism responsible for silkworm disease.

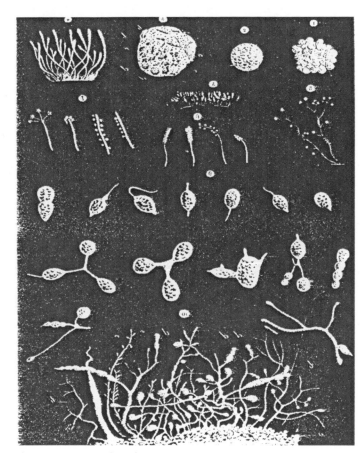

Figure 11.2. Continued.

lowing any use of surgery. It is to the credit of Joseph Lister to have mounted a major movement to utilize antiseptic chemicals for the cleaning of instruments and for the washing of hands to reduce the number of infections that could be transmitted from one patient to another.

Bassi's silkworm studies were recorded in two writings in 1835 and 1836—one entitled *Theoretical Part* and the other called *Practical Part*.

Twenty-seven years after Bassi had presented his silkworm studies supporting the basic concepts of the origin of infectious diseases, Pasteur was able to successfully repeat Bassi's research investigations for silkworm disease and reaffirm the parasitic origin of infectious diseases.

The studies of Bassi and the clear and definitive experiments that he performed, as well as the conclusions that he made from these years of research on diseases of the silkworm and infectious diseases of other organisms, permitted him to elucidate the general theory that microorganisms cause infectious diseases.

A more recent report by Renata Ferreira and Robert Martins, (1997) in reviewing the studies of Agostino Bassi, concluded that Bassi's research: ". . . was the first case in which the causal connection between a microorganism and a disease was established by experiment."

Even France, despite the well-known research efforts of Louis Pasteur, recognized the significant contributions of Bassi and awarded him the title of Knight of the Legion of Honor. Bassi was awarded diplomas from academies in many countries. He was awarded gold and silver medals from several countries. However, he was obliged to melt many of these medals to procure funds that he required to continue his work and also to provide funds to help some of his friends and relatives.

Bassi's work was appreciated by many scholars throughout the world, but primarily in Italy (Bajla, 1923; Baroni, *et al.* 1924; Belloni, *et al.* (1956); Calandruccio, 1892; Capparoni, 1894; Dossena, 1954; Faucci, 1936, 1937, 1939, and 1941; Grassi, 1925; Petenghi, 1856; Redaelli, *et al.* 1939).

Bassi's research and his studies with the organism infecting the silkworms, *Beauveria bassiana,* may have a major impact on the reduction of malaria infections, because his organism has now been shown to be lethal to the *Anopheles* mosquito which insect transmits the largest number of malaria infections to humans. (*The Scientist*, Vol. 23 No. 10, October 2009, pp. 44–50)

Having expended his energies and his money, and being nearly totally blind, Bassi died in February of 1856.

Bassi was buried in a tomb in the Church of Saint Francis in the square of the Ospedale Vecchio in Lodi, Italy, next to the two famous poets of Lodi, Francesco Da Lemene and Ada Negri.

NOTES

1. It is now a generally accepted practice in hospitals and other healthcare institutions that every room where a patient is examined has mounted near the Exit Door an inverted dispenser of a disinfectant. Every individual who leaves that room and has had contact with a patient procures a few drops of the disinfectant and rubs their hands together to ensure that transmission of any organisms from one patient to another is not carried by the healthcare individual.

2. See Giacomo Barbo, 1836.

3. "Sie kennen ohne Zweifel Bassi's schöne Entdeckung über die wahre Natur der Muscardine. Die Thatsache scheint mir von höchstem Interesse fur die Pathogenie, obgleich meines Wissens auch nicht ein Arzt sie bisher seiner Aufmerksamkeit gewürdigt hatte. Ich liess mir deshalb zahlreiche Exemplare von Seidenwürmern, die an der Muscardine litten, von Mailand kommen, und meine damit angestellten Versuche haben nicht bloss Bassi's und Audouin's Angaben bestätigt, sondern noch einige audere nicht ganz unwichtige Resultate ergeben."

Bibliography

Alfieri, E. "Bollet. della Soc. Medico-chirurgica di Pavia". Verbali delle Adunanze, Seduta, Anno XXXV, N. 6, p. 823, 12 Gennaìo 1923.

Alfieri, Maragnoli, Bertarelli, Cicardi, Riquier, Baldi, Perroncito, Montemartini, Bajla. "L'avvenire del disinfettatore" Numero Unico. Lanzani, Milano 1924.

American Public Health Association, Inc. *Standard Methods for the Examination of Dairy Products,* 1997.

Archarbe, Gazeppa (Enrico). Practical Theoretical Doctrine, 1822.

Bajla, E. *Agostino Bassi di Lodi* (1773–1856). Il vero fondatore della teoria parassitaria delle infezioni e precursore di Pasteur. In 8, pp. 15. (Estratto dal "Bollettino dell'Ordine dei Medici." Anno X. N. 12. Milano, Tip. Cordani (Bibl. Laudense: XXIV. C. 237) 1923.

———. *Agostino Bassi di Lodi.* Il vero fondatore della teoria parassitaria delle infezioni e precursore di Pasteur. "Giornale della Società Italiana d'Igiene" Anno XLVI, fasc. 2. Tip. Fossati. Milano 1924. (a)

———. *Il fondatore della teoria parassitaria delle infezioni. Agostino Bassi di Lodi.* Da "La Medicina Italiana" N. 3, Milano, 31 Marzo, 1924. (b)

Bajlo, J. *Uno sguardo alla Bachicultura trivigiana nel passato e Agostino Bassi.* Da "Il contadino della Marca Trivigiana" Treviso, Giugno 1924.

Barbò, conte Giacomo (Jacques). *De La Muscardine (Maladie des Ders à soie).* Paris, Chez Les Principaux Libraires, 1836.

Baroni, G. *A. Bassi nel terzo cinquantenario della nasita.* "Il Cittadino" Lodi, 9 Febbraio 1924.

Baroni, Giovanni, Besana, Carlo, Talini, Bassano. *Comune di Lodi. In onore di Agostino Bassi.* Ottobre 1924. Lodi, Tip. Biancardi. In 8, pp. 47, fig. (Bibl. Laudense: XXIV. C.240)—1924

Balbiani, Edouard-Gérard. *Compt. Rend. Acd. D. Sc.* Paris, t. CIII, p. 952. 1886.

Bassi, Agostino. *Breve cenno sulla moltiplicazione e migliorazione delle pecore no. strane cogli Arieli spagnuoli.* p. 8; (Lodi?), Veladini, s. d. (Per la data cfr. il testo a p. 3). in 24—(1808).

155

————. *Della pastorizia e della più utile coltura dei pomi di terra. (La controcopertina porta invece per titolo*: Il pastore ben istruilo). p. 482; sei tabelle nel testo; due tavole incise in rame in fine del volume; Milano, Destefanis, in 8 (Precedono: lettera dedicatoria I–VI; Prefazione VII–XVI; Prospetto dell-opera XVII–XXIV)— 1812.

————. *Dell'utilità ed uso del pomo di terra e del metodo migliore di coltivarlo.* p. 47; Lodi, Pallavicini, in 8—1817.

————. *Osservazioni sull'opera del sovescio e nuovo sistema fertilizzante senza dispendio di concio.* p. 50; Lodi, Pallavicini, in 8—1819.

————. *sulla fabbrica del formaggio all'uso lodigiano.* p. 22; Lodi, Orcesi, in 8 (Prima che dall' Orcesi questo lavoro, al dire dello stesso Bassi, è stato stampato nel 1820 dal Lamperti in Milano; di questa edizione non si trovano esemplari). L'opuscolo posseduto dalla Comunale di Lodi porta una dedica autografa del Bassi al Dott. Fisico Enrico Morandini 1820.

————. *Lettera sui paragrandini.* p. 11; Milano, Brambilla, (L'opuscolo posseduto dalla Comunale di Lodi presenta alle pp. 5, 6, 8 e 9 correzioni a penna molto probabilmente del Bassi).

————. *Memoria sui nuovi metodi di vinificazionè.* p. 42' (Con una tavola incisa in rame in fine dell' opuscolo); Lodi, Orcesi, 1823; in 8. Recensito in Biblioteca italiana. Tomo 32, pp. 78 e 333. A p. 336 è riportata uno lettera del Bassi al recensore in data 14-XII-1823.

————. *Nuova maniera di fabbricare il vino a tino coperto senza l' uso di alcuna macchina.* p. 46; Lodi, Orcesi, in 8—1824.

————. *Analisi critica dei quattro discorsi del conte Carlo Verri intorno al vino ed alla vite.* p. 71; Milano, Rusconi, in 8—1824.

————. *Nuova maniera di fabbricare il vino a tino coperlo ecc.* Ediz. II., riveduta ed ampliata, p. 48; Lodi, Orcesi, in 8—1825.

————. *Nuovi cenni intorno all'arte di fabbricare i vini, all'educazione dei filugelli e dei mori ed altri oggetti agrari.* p. 24; Lodi, Orcesi, in 8—1826.

————. *Del mal del segno, calcinaccio o moscardino, malattia che affligge i bachi da seta e sul modo di liberarne le bigattaie anche le più infestate.* Parte I, Teorica, p. I–IX, 1–67; Lodi, Orcesi, in 8 1835.

————. *Id. Parte II, Pratica.* p. I–XIV, 1–58; Lodi, Orcesi, in 8—1836.

————. *Memoria in addizione all' opera sul Calcino.* p. 38; Milano, Molina, marzo, in 8° (In appendice sono riportate (p. 24) le relazioni dei vantaggi ottenuti da bachicultori coi metodi del Bassi) 1837.

————. *Del mal del segno ecc.* Parte Teorica e Pratica; IIa Edizione riveduta, corretta ad accresciuta, p. 112; Milano, Molina, maggio; in 8—1837.

————. *Memoria in addizione all' opera sul Calcino.* p. 40; Milano, Molina, maggio in 8 (In appendice (p.24) ancora le relazioni predette). [Delle tre opere sul Calcino pare (Briosi) siano state fatte edizioni anche a Novara ed a Torino]—1837.

————. *Breve istruzione per evitare il danno che reca il Calcino ecc.* p. 42; Milano, Molina, 1839; in 8. (Contiene inoltre (p. 43–63) un indirizzo del Bassi ai bachicultori ed alcune relazioni degli stessi).

————. Tre nuove memorie sui gelsi (p. 1–25), sui vini (p. 27–40), e sui contagi (p. 41–57). p. 57; Lodi, Wilmant, 1844; in 8°. (Nello stesso anno le tre memorie furono dal Wilmant stampate separatamente coi seguenti titoli: Sui contagi in generale a specialmente su quelli che affliggono l' umana specie. Dei Gelsi ed in specie intorno al modo di prevenire, scoprire e curare la Gangrena che fa perire gran numero di quesli alberi preziosi. Il miglior melodo di fare e conservare lungamente i vini).

————. *Il vero e l' utile nella educazione dei filugelli e dei gelsi.* p. 55; Lodi, Wilmant, in 8,1845.

————. *Discorsi sulla natura e cura della pellagra.* p. 35; Milano, Chiusi, in 8. Da p. 26–35 si trovano: a) Sulla malattia che attaccò i pomi di terra e come si possa arrestarla; b) Rimedi sicuri e pronti contro le febbri intermittenti; c) Rimedio contro le scottature; d) Rimedio contro le inflammazioni degli occhi, 1846.

————. *Studí sul Calcino dei bachi da seta.* p. 8; Milano, Bernardoni, 1848; in 8. Estratto dall' Eco della Borsa, 23, II, 1848.

————. *Osservazioni sugli studí dei signori Guerin-Meneville ed Eugenio Robert intorno al Calcino.* p. 29; Milano, Redaelli, in 8, 1849.

————. *Istruzioni per prevenire e curare il Colera asiatico.* p. 42; Lodi, Wilmant, in 8, 1849.

————. *Il fatto parlante all'Autore sul modo di ben governare i bachi da seta nonchè su quello di prevenire e curare il terribile Calcino.* p. 45; Lodi, Wilmant, in 8, 1850.

————. *Addizione al fatto parlante.* ¼ di foglio in 8, senz' altra segnatura. (Stampata due mesi dopo il lavoro precedente, 1850).

————. *Il miglior governo dei bachi da seta.* p. 78; Lodi, Wilmant, in 16, 1851.

————. *Appendice al miglior governo.* p. 9; Lodi, Wilmant, in 16, 1851.

————. *Della più utile coltivazione dei bachi da seta.* p. 108; Lodi, Wilmant, 1851; in 16. (La materia nelle tre monografie (ai n. 24, 26 e 28) è fondamentalmente identica, solo vi è distribuita con qualche variante, soppressione od aggiunta. Le tre monografie mirano alla volgarizzazione delle nozioni teoriche e pratiche stabilite dal Bassi e sopratutto a far emanare dall'Autorità norme profilattiche e curative contro il Calcino).

— —. *Piccola memoria addizionale alla più utile coltivazione dei bachi da seta.* ¼ di foglio in 16, senz' altra segnatura (1851).

————. *Dei parassiti generatori dei contagi.* p. 28; Lodi, Wilmant, 1851; in 16.

————. *Istruzioni sicure per liberare le uve dalla malattia dominante.* p. 8 Lodi, Wilmant, 1852; in 16.

————. *Della natura dei morbi ossia mali contagiosi e del modo di prevenirli e curarli.* p. 8; Lodi, Wilmant, 1853; in 16.

————. *Societa Medico Chirurgica di Pavia.* 1925. Opere di Agostino Bassi, p. 673 and lxviii. Tapografia Cooperativa di Pavia.

Bellinzona, Ing. Giuseppe. Lodi attraverso il secolo XIX (A. Bassi a pp. 8–9, 24–27) Marinoni, Lodi 1901.

Belloni, Luigi, Letizia Vergnano, and Attilio Zambianchi. *Studi Su A. Bassi.* Archivio Storico Lodigiano, 1956.

————. *Documenti Bassiana*, Per IL LVII Congresso Della Societa Italiana Di Medicina Interna E IL LVIII Congresso Della Societa Italiana Di Chirurgia (Milano—15–18 Ottobre 1956).

Benedicenti, A. *Malati, Medici e Farmacisti*. Hcepli, Milano 1925.

Bern, Switzerland pamphlet reprinted in the "Rec. de méd. Vét., p. 624, Paris 1886.

Bertarelli, E. *Un precursore di Pasteur. Agostino Bassi*. "Il Secolo" Milano, 26 Gennaio 1924. (a)

————. *Agostino Bassi* (1773–1856). Commemorazione tenuta alla Società Medica di Pavia il, Succ. Bruni e Marelli, Pavia, 2 Maggio 1924. (b)

Besana. *In Memoria di Agostino Bassi*. "Archivio storico per la città di Lodi". Anno 42, 1923.

Bizzarini, G. *Agostino Bassi*. Conferenza tenuta all' Università del Popolo "Giosuè Carducci" il, in Livorno 27 Aprile 1924. (a)

————. *Per la rivendicazione di un diritto italiano di priorità. Agostino Bassi*. Dal Giornale "Il Telegrafo" di Livorno, Febbraio 1924. (b)

Brambilla, Elena. Wien, Haus-Hof-end Staatsarchiv, Italienisch-Spanischer Rat; Lombardei Collectanea + Lomb. Coll. Microfilmed in theArchives of the State of Milan, 1982.

————. "Il 'sistema letterario' di Milano. Professioni nobili e professioni borghesi dall' eta spagnola alle riforme teresiane", in A. DE MADDALENA, E. ROTELLI, AND G. BARBARISI, eds., *Economia, istituzioni, cultura in Lombardia nell'eta di Maria Teresa, 3 vols., Bologna, 1982.*

Brannigan, Augustine. *The Social Basis of Scientific Discoveries*. New York: Cambridge University Press, 1981.

Briosi. *Cenno biografico di Agostino Bassi*. "Atti del R. Istituto Botanico dell'Università di Pavia". Nuova serie, Vol. VIII, 1904.

Brock, Thomas. "Pasteur: High Priest of Microbiology" American Society of Microbiology News, Vol. 61, No. 11, 1995.

Calandruccio, Salvatore. *Agostino Bassi di Lodi il Fondatore della Teoria Parassitaria e delle cure parassiticide*. Martinez, Catania. (a) In 8, pp. 75. (Bibl. Laudense : XXIV. C. 233), 1892.

————. *Aggiunte dell' Autobiografia del Bassi*. "Archives de Parasitologie" Tomo VI, p. 42. 1902. (b)

Capparoni, Pietro. Per la prioritàdi una rivendicazione. Agostino Bassi ricordato dal Professore G. Martinotti fin dal quale 1894 quale fondatore della teoria parassitaria delle infezioni. In: «Bollettino dell'Istituto Storico Italiano dell'Arte sanitaria», vol. 5, pp. 231–232, 1925.

Cassier, Maurice. "Studies in History and Philosophy of Science." Biomedical Sciences, Volume 36, Issue 4, December 2005.

Chamberland, Charles E. British Patent Number 25,606 issued in 1902 entitled "Improvements in Filters."

————. British Patent Number 27,180 issued in 1905 entitled "Improvements in and relating to Filters for Water and other Liquids."

————. British Patent Number 16,270 issued in 1911 entitled "Improvements in and relating to Filters and Filtering Apparatus."

Charrin. *Compt. Rend. Soc. De biol.*, Paris, 1889, pp. 250, 330, 627; and pp. 203, 332, 195—1890.

Cicardi, F. *A proposito di Agostino Bassi e Luigi Pasteur.* L' "Unione" di Lodi, N. 44, 29 Ottobre 1924. Succ. Wilmant, Lodi, e "Il Policlinico" fasc. 38, 1924.

Clerici, A. *Un precursore Italiano di Luigi Pasteur (A. Bassi).* "Corriere della Sera" Milano del 26 Settembre, 1923.

Cogrossi, Carlo Francesco. *Nuova Idea Del Male Contagioso De' Buo.i* published in Milan 1714.

Crivelli, Balsamo. *Osservazioni sopra una nuova specie di mucedinea del genere "Botrylis" che si svolge sopra i bachi da seta e le crisalidi morte di calcino; indagini riguardo alla sua origine.* In "Bibl. Ital." LXXIX, Milano p. 125, 1835.

———. *Aufstellung von zwei neuen Arten Mucedineen, Botrylis Bassiana und Mucor radicans, und über die Entwicklung der ersteren Arten in Seidenwurme.* "Linnaea" X, p. 609, 1835–1836.

———. *Sopra l'origine e lo sviluppo della "Botrylis Bassiana" e sopra una specie di Mucorino, anch'esso parassito.* "Bibl. Ital." XV p. 367, Milano, 1838.

———. *Ueber der Ursprung und die Entwicklung der "Botrylis Bassiana" und einere andere schmarotzende Art von Schimmel.* "Linnaea" XIII, p. 118, 1839.

———. *Agostino Bassi. Nuovo cenno.* "Gazzetta dello Provincia di Lodi e Crema" N. 7 del 16 Febbraio 1856.

D'Hérelle, F. *Le Bactériophage et ses Applications ThéThe Bacteriophage and its Therapeutic Applications.* OCLC 14749145.

Debrè, Patrice. *Louis Pasteur* (translated by Elborg Forster), The Johns Hopkins University Press 1998.

Donitz. *Die Deutsche Klinik am Eingange des XX Jahrhundert.* Urban u. Schwarzenberg, Wien, 1901.

Dossena, Gaetano. *Quello che la medicina deve ad Agostino Bassi.* In: «Archivio storico lodigiano». Serie II, anno II, gennaio 1954, pp. 41–55. (Bibl. Braidense: Per. IV. 1). 1954.

Dubos, René. *Louis Pasteur: Free Lance of Science*—Boston: Little, Brown & Co. 1950.

Farley, J., and G. L. Geison. *Science, politics and spontaneous generation in nineteenth century France: The Pasteur-Pouchet debate.* Bull. Hist. Med. 48:161–198, 1974.

Faucci, Ugo. *In memoria di Agostino Bassi (1773–1856) (Nel I Centenario del ". . . Mal del segno").* In: "Rivista di Storia delle Scienze Mediche e Naturali," 1936, 18, anno XXVII, pp. 1–26, 59–102, 153–206, 286–326; 371–428; 1937, 19, anno XXVIII, pp. 24–27, 283–305; 1939, 21, anno XXX, pp. 85–98, 209–228; 23, anno XXXII, pp. 1–32. (Bibl. Nazionale, Firenze). 1941.

Ferraretto, *T. Agostino Bassi, alunno. Il suo microscopio nel Laboratorio di Fisica.* Liceo-Ginnasio P. Verri di Lodi. Succ. Wilmant, Lodi, 1924.

Federico, P. J. "Louis Pasteur's Patents" Science, Volume 86, p. 327, October 8, 1937.

Ferreira, Renata Rivera, and Robert de Andrade Martins. *Primórdios da moderna teoria dos germes: Agostino Bassi e a doença dos bichos-da-seda. Epistéme. Filosofia e*

História das Ciências em Revista or Philosophy and History of Sciences in Magazine 2(3):55–71, 1997.

Findlen, Paula. *Possessing Nature.* University of California Press, 1994.

Freudenreich, E. Von. *Bakteriologische Untersuchungen über den Reifungsprozess des Emmenthaler Käses. Landwirthsch. Jahrb.* Der Schweiz. 1891.

———. *De la perméabilité des filters Chamberland à l'égard des Bactéries.* Ann. De micrographie. IV. 1891–92.

———. *Ueber die Durchlässigkeit der Chamberlandfilter für Bakterien.* Centralbl. F. Bakt. U. Paras. XII. 1892.

Geison, Gerald L. *The Private Science of Louis Pasteur.* Princeton University Press, 1995.

Grassi, G. B. *I progressi della Biologia e delle sue applicazioni pratiche consequiti in Italia nell'ultimo cinquantennio.* "Cinquant'anni di Storia Italiana" Vol. III., a cura dell'Accademia dei Lincei, Hoepli, Milano 1911.

———. *Agostino Bassi precursore di Luigi Pasteur, di Roberto Koch e di Giuseppe Lister.* Dalla "Difesa Sociale" Anno III., N.2, Roma 1924.

———. *Commentario all'opera parassitologica (sui contagi) di Agostino Bassi.* In: Bassi Agostino "Opere . . .," anno XXIX, pp. 251–259. aprile 1956.

Gruber, M. *Ueber die Methoden der Prüfung der Desinfektionsmittel.* VII. Intern. Congr. F. Hygiene and demography, London, 1891.

———. Centralbl. Für Bakt. U. Parasitenk. XI. 1892.

Hansen, E. Chr. *Les champignons stercoraires du Danemark.* Résumé d'un mémoire publié dans les "Videnskbl. Meddelelser" de la Société d'histoire naturelle de Copenhague. 1876.

———. Contributions à la connaissance des organismes qui peuvent se trouver dans la bière et le moût de bière et y vivre. *Compt. Rend. des Meddel.* fra Carlsberg Laboratoriet. I., 2. Copenhagen, 1879.

Häser, H. "Lehrbuch der Geschichte der Medicin," 3te Aufl., Jean, 1881, Bd. II S. 1075.

Hume, Ethel Douglas. *Pasteur Exposed. Germs-Genes-Vaccines.* Bookreal, 1923.

Ingras, G. A. *Agostino Bassi.* "Il Policlinico" Sezione Pratica, Fasc. 36, p. 1178, Roma 1923.

Jörgensen, Alfred. *Micro-Organisms and Fermentation.* Macmillan and Co., Limited. 1900.

Koch, R. *Ueber Desinfektion.* Mitt. D. K. Gesundheitsamtes. 1881.

———. *Zur Untersuchung von pathogenen Organismen.* Mitt. d. K. Gesundheitsamtes. I. Berlin, 1881.

Koen, J.S. "A Practical Method for Field Diagnosis of Swine Disease" *American Journal of Veterinarian Medicine.* 14: 468, 1919.

Kohn, Alexander. *False Prophets.* Basil Blackwell, Ltd. Oxford, UK, 1986.

Kovalevsky. Bull. Acad. *D. sc. De St Petersb.,* t. XIII, p. 437, 1894.

Lanctôt, Ghislaine Saint-Pierre. *The Medical Mafia*—Ghislaine Saint-Pierre Lanctôt, Waterloo, Canada, 1994.

Lastrucci, Carlo L. *The Scientific Approach: Basic Principles of the Scientific Method,* Massachusetts: Schenkman Publishing Company, Inc., 1963.

Leclerc, Yvan. "Pasteur, Cahiers D'un Savant" Publiee avec la cooperation scientifique de l'ITEM-CNRS et la collaboration de la Bibliotheque Nationale de France, page 113 of Pasteur's notebook 108, 1995.

Lombroso, C. Prefazione alla ristampa dei "Discorsi di A. Bassi sulla natura e cura della Pellagra" Torino, Bocca 1903.

Lomeni, Dott. Ignazio. *L'innocuita e L'efficacia, De' Liscivi Medicinali, Proposti— Dal Sig. Dott. Di Leggi Agostino Bassi Di Lodi.* Milano Presso la Società degli Editori degli Annali Universali delle Scienze e dell' Industria Nella Galleria Decristoforis Sopra Lo Scalone A Sinistra, 1836.

Maddox, Brenda. *Rosalind Franklin-The Dark Lady of DNA.* HarperCollins Publishers, 2002.

Marenduzzo, A. *Prefazione accompagnatoria ai Presidi dei Licei ed Istituti d'Italia di "A. Bassi di Lodi" del Prof. E. Bajla.* Milano, Cordani 1923.

McNeil, Donald G. Jr. cited from The New York Times. June 10, 2005.

Mesnil. *Ann. De l'Inst. Pasteur*, t. IX, p. 301, Paris, 1895.

Metchnikoff, Elie. *Diseases of the larvae of the grain weevil. Insects harmful to agriculture (series) Issue III.* The Grain Weevil, (in Russian), Odessa, USSR, pp. 32, 1879.

———. *Virchow's Archiv*, Berlin, Bd. XCVII, S. 502, 1884.

———. *Immunity in Infectious Diseases.* Cambridge: The University Press, 1905.

Mieli. *Agostino Bassi.* "Archivio di storia della Scienza" N. 1, Roma 1924.

Monti, A. *I dati fondamentali della patologia moderna.* Rosenberg e Sellier, Torino (Questa opera é stata tradotta in inglese dall'Eyre e pubblicata a Londra nel 1900 a cura della Sydenam Society) 1898.

Morbidity and Mortality Weekly Report (Centers for Disease Control and Prevention) *Escherichia coli* O157:H7 'Infection Associated with Drinking Raw Milk' Washington and Oregon, November—December 2005,/ 56(08); 265–267. March 2, 2007.

Morens, David M., Gregory Folkers, and Anthony Fauci. Hektoen International, A Journal of Healthcare, Humanities, and Medical History, "Emerging Infections: A Perpetual Challenge" Lancet, Volume 8, Issue 11, pp 710–719, November 2008.

Oeuvres, VI, pp. 358–369

Oldrini, G. Archivio Storico di Lodi. La Biblioteca Laudense. Agostino Bassi Bibliotecario. Borini, Lodi 1921.

———. *Storia della Cultura laudense.* pp. 380–387, 1885.

Pasteur, Louis. *Etudes sur la maladie des vers a soie.* Gautheir-Villars, Paris, Vol. I., p. 22, 1870.

———. The Physiological Theory of Fermentation, presented to the Academy of Sciences April 10th and 24th, 1876.

———. Examen du rôle attribué au gaz oxygène atmosphérique dans la destruction des matières animales et végétales après la mort; par M.L. Pasteur. In: "C.R. de l'Académie des Sciences," 56, pp. 734–740. (Ist. Lombardo: R. III.56). 1863.

———. United States Patent 135,245 'Brewing Beer and Ale' patented—1873.

———. United States Patent 141,072 claiming a 'yeast, free from organic germs of diseases, as an article of manufacture.' 1873.

Pasteur, L., Joubert, Jules, and Charles Chamberland. La theorie des germes et ses applications a la medicine et a la chirurgie. Comptes Rendus Hebdomadaires des Seances de l'Academie des Sciences. 86:1037–1043, 1878.

Petenghi, Mosè. Cenni intorno alla vita ed alle opera del Dott. Agostino Bassi. Lodi, C. Wilmant e Figli. In 8, pp. 22 nn. (R9istampa dell'opera precede3nte) (Bibl. Laudense: XXIV. C. 232). 1856.

———. Cenni intorno alla vita ed alle opere del Dottor Agostino Bassi, in "Gazzetta della Provincia di Lodi e Crema" N. 15 del 12 Aprile 1856.

Porter, J. R. Agostino Bassi Bicentennial (1773–1973) Bacteriological Reviews, Vol. 37, No. 3, p.284–288 1973.

Procacci, Giuliano. *History of the Italian People*. Cox & Wyman Ltd, London, 1968.

Redaelli, P. and V. Visocchi. "Agostino Bassi precursor of comparative mycopathology" *Mycopathologia* 2:37–42, 1939.

Redi, Francesco. *Esperienze intorno* alla generazione degl'insetti fatted a Francesco Redi . . . e da lui scritte in una lettera all'illustrissimo Signor Carlo Dati. Firenze, all'Insegna della Stella, 1668. In 8, pp. 228, fig, tavv. 28. (Bibl. Braidense, ZNN. IV. 4).

———. Osservazioni di Francesco Redi . . . intorno agli animali viventi che si trovano negli animali viventi. Firenze, Piero Matini, 1684. In 8, pp. 4 nn., 232, tavv. 26. (Bibl. Braidense, D. XII. 10833).

Riquier, Giuseppe Carlo. Per Agostino Bassi nel III cinquantenario della sua nascita (26 settembre 1773—8 febbraio 1856) Proposta di ristampa e diffusione delle sue opere. Pavia, Tip. Cooperativa, 1923. In 8, pp. 17. (Estratto dal Bollettino della Società Medico-Chirurgica di Pavia, anno XXXV, fasc. 4, 1923). (Bibl. Laudense : XXIV. C. 236). 1923.

———. *A. Bassi, fondatore della teoria microbica ed antisettica*. Da "Il Popolo d'Italia" Milano 23 November 1923. (a)

———. Per Agostino Bassi nel terzo cinquantenario della sua nascita. Proposta di ristampa e diffusione delle sue Opere. "Bollettino della Società Medico-chirurgica di Pavia". Anno XXXV, fasc. 4, 1923, e "Archivio storico per la Città di Lodi". Anno 42, 1923. (b)

———. Per il III Cinquantenario della nascita di Agostino Bassi (1773–1856). Commemorazione tenuta dal Prof. Dott. Giuseppe Carlo Riquier in occasione dello scoprimento di una lapide al Bassi nel Minicipio di Mairago il 18 Novembre 1923. Lodi, Tip. Borini-Abbiati, 1924. In 8, pp. 15. (Estratto dall'Archivio Storico Lodigiano, anno XLII.).—(Bibl. Laudense: XXIV. C. 238). 1924.

———. *Agostino Bassi nel terzo cinquantenario della sua nascita*. Commemorazione tenuta in occasione dello scoprimento di una lapide al Bassi nel Municipio di Mairago, il 18 Novembre 1923. Tip. Popolare, Pavia 1924. (c)

———. Agostino Bassi fondatore della teoria microbica ed antisettica. "Rivista di storia delle Scienze Mediche" Anno XV, N. 1–2, 1924. (d)

———. *Agostino Bassi e la sua Opera*. Commemorazione ufficiale tenuta alla R. Università di Sassari. Tip. Cooperativa, Pavia 1924. (e)

Sambon. "Pasteur and his work historically considered." *Journal of Tropical Medicine* 15, V. 1923.

Schwann. *Vorläufige Mitteilung betreffend Versuche über die Weingärung und Fäulnis.* Poggend. Ann. XLI. 1837.

Sanarelli, G. Agostino Bassi. Prolusione al corso di perfezionamento in Igiene per gli Ufficiali Sanitari. "Il Policlinico" Roma, fasc. 8, 1924.

Silva, Bernardino. Agostino Bassi, Fondatore della teoria parassitaria e parassiticida od antisettica. 1773–1856. Commemorazione letta a Lodi Tip. Dell'Avo. il 26 Settembre 1901.

———. Agostino Bassi fondatore della teoria parassitaria e parassiticida od antisettica. 1773–1856. Commemorazione letta a Lodi il 26 Settembre 1901 dal Dott. Prof. B. Silva . . . Lodi, C. Dell'Avo, In 8, pp. 56. (Bibl. Laudense : XXIV. C. 234). 1901.

Silvetti, A.N. Polysaccharides as Effective Chemo-attractants to White Blood Cells and Macrophages. Federation Proc. (46 A3868) 980, 1987.

———. "Mechanisms Involved in Wound Healing." Faseb Journal (3–A5956) A1251, 1993.

Smith, Kendall A. "Wanted, an Anthrax Vaccine: Dead or Alive." from Med Immunol. 2005; 4:5.

Spallanzani, Lazzaro. *Propositiones physico-mathematicae.* Reggio Emilia, 1757.

———. *Riflessioni intorno alla traduzione dell'Iliade del Salvini* . . . Parma 1760.

———. *Saggio di osservazioni microscopiche concernenti il sistema della generazione dei Signori de Needham e Buffon.* In his *Dissertazione due* . . . Modena, 1765.

———. *Memorie sopre I muli.* . . . On sterility in hybrids. Modena, 1768.

———. *Dell'azione del cuore.* . . . On the circulation of the blood. Modena, 1768.

———. *Prodromo di un opera da imprimersi sopra la riproduzioni animali.* Modena, 1768.

———. *De' fenomeni della circolazione osservata nel giro universale de' vasi etc.* On the circulation in cold-blooded animals and chick embryos. Modena 1773.

French translation by Joseph Tourdes (1770–1851) as *Expériences sur la circulation.* . . . Paris, 1800.

English translation R. Hall as: *Experiments upon the Circulation of the Blood.* London, 1801.

———. *Opuscoli di fiscia animale e vegetabile.* 2 volumes. Modena, Soc. Tipografica, 1776.

French translation by Jean Senebier as: *Opuscules de physique, animale, et végétabile.* 2 volumes, Geneva, 1777, 1785, 1786, 1787.

English translation by Thomas Beddoes (1754–1808) as: *Tracts on Animals and Vegetables.* 2 volumes, London, 1784, 1786.

English translation by J. Dalyell: *Tracts on the Nature of Animals and Vegetables.* 2 volumes, Edinburgh, 1799.

Second edition as: *Tracts on the Natural History of Animals and Vegetables.* Edinburgh, 1803.

Later confutation of the theory of spontaneous generation. Spallanzani's conclusions were similar to those expressed by Pasteur's nearly a century later.

———. *Expériences sur la digestion de l'homme et de différentes espèces d'animaux* . . . Geneva, 1783, 1784; facsimile edition, Paris, 1756. *Expériences pour servir à l'histoire de la génération des animaux et des plantes* . . . Geneva, 1785.

————. *Fecondazione artificiale di una cagna.* Opusculi scelti sulle scienze e sulli ati . . . 1781, 4: 279–282.

————. *Viaggi alle due Sicilie e in alcune parti dell'Appennino.* 6 volumes in 8, Pavia, B. Comini, 1792–1797.

French translation: *Voyages dans les Deux-Siciles, et dans quelques parties des Apennins.* 6 volumes. Bern, 1795–1797.

German translation: *Des Abtes Spallanzani Reisen in beyde Sicilien und in Gegenden der Appenninen.* 5 volumes. Leipzig, 1795. 1798.

English translation: *Travels in the two Silicies, and some parts of the Apennines.* 4 volumes. London, 1798.

————. *Lettere sul volo dei pipistrelli acciecati.* Giornale de letterati, 13: 120–186, 1974.

————. *Lettera scritta dal sig. Lazzaro* (sic) *Spallanzani.* di Modena sotto di 25 Maggio 1766 al sig. Abate Fontana professore pubblico dell'Università di Pisa dimorante in Firenze. In: "Continuazione delle Novelle Letterarie" Firenze, n., 46, 15 Novembre 1766 coll. 722–725. (Bibl. Braidense: ZF. 8.46). 1766.

————. *Lettera del sig. Ab. Lazzaro Spallanzani.* al sig. Felice Fontana, che contiene un'osservazione assai bella intorno gli Animalculi delle infusioni. In: "Giornale d'Italia spettante alla scienza naturale" T. III, Venezia, Milocco, pp. 12–13. (Bibl. Braidense: ZEE. III. 20). 1767(a).

————. Progetto del celebre sig. Needham intorno a cui brama che ne sia informato il Pubblico. In: "Giornale d'Italia spettante alla scienza naturale" Tomo III, Venezia, Milocco, pp. 409–411. (Bibl. Braidense, ZEE. III.20). 1767 (b).

————. De' Fenomeni della circolazione Osservata nel giro universale de' Vasi; De' fenomeni della circolazione languente; De' moti del sangue independenti dall'azione del cuore; e del pulsar delle arterie. Dissertazioni quattro dell'Abate Spallanzi . . . Modena, Società Tipografica. In 8, pp. VIII, 343, 1 nn., tav. 1. (Bibl. Braidense, A. II. 222). 1773.

Strick, James E. "New Details Add to Our Understanding of Spontaneous Generation Controversies." American Society for Microbiology News, Volume 63, Number 4, pp.193–198, 1997.

————. The British spontaneous generation debates of 1860–1880: medicine, evolution and laboratory science in the Victorian context. Ph.D. dissertation, Princeton University, Princeton, N.J. 1997.

Talini, B. *Proposta di Onoranze ad Agostino Bassi.* Dell'Avo, Lodi 1901.

Talini, B., C. Besana, and G. Baroni. *Lodi per Agostino Bassi.* Biancardi, Lodi 1924.

Trambusti. *Luigi Pasteur.* Zanichelli, Bologna 1923.

Vallery-Radot, Pasteur. *Louis Pasteur: A Great Life in Brief.* Trans. Alfred Joseph. New York: Knopf, 1958.

Veritas. Giornale "La Sera" del 20 Settembre, Milano 1923.

Von Behring and Nissen. *Ztschr. F. Hyg., Leipzig,* 1890, Bd. VIII, S. 412.

Weston A. Price Foundation. Web:www.westonaprice.org "A Campaign for Real Milk" PMB 106-380, 4200 Wisconsin Avenue, NW, Washington DC 20016.

About the Author

The author, **George H. Scherr,** was born in New York City in 1920. He received a B.S. degree from Queens College in 1941. He also earned M.S. and Ph.D. degrees from the University of Kentucky in 1949 and 1951, respectively. While serving in the U.S. Army during World War II, he worked in the Biological Warfare unit at Fort Detrick, MD.

Scherr has published more than 100 papers primarily concerned with infectious diseases. He was Assistant Professor of Microbiology at the Creighton University School of Medicine and Associate Tenured Professor at the University of Illinois School of Medicine.

For 40 years, he was the editor and publisher of the *Journal of Irreproducible Results*, a magazine of science humor and satire.

Scherr holds over 100 patents in over 25 countries. He synthesized for the first time the molecule silver alginate, which has been shown to have the properties of being lethal to a broad array of microorganisms with no result of resistance. The silver alginate is also lethal to a number of viruses, molds, and yeasts. It has been incorporated into medical dressings for the treatment of infected lesions and burns in over 120 countries.

CPSIA information can be obtained at www.ICGtesting.com
Printed in the USA
BVOW040930151111

276098BV00002B/5/P